The Ultimate Autoimmune Solution

A Revolutionary Plan to Prevent and Reverse Autoimmune Diseases

Dr EMILY JOHN

COPYRIGHT PAGE

TABLE OF CONTENTS

INTRODUCTION

utoimmune diseases are a complex and growing concern in modern medicine. They are characterized by an overactive immune system that attacks healthy cells, tissues, and organs in the body, causing a range of chronic health conditions. The exact causes of autoimmune diseases are not well understood, but they are believed to be related to genetic, environmental, and lifestyle factors.

According to the National Institute of Allergy and Infectious Diseases, there are more than 80 different types of autoimmune diseases, including rheumatoid arthritis, lupus, multiple sclerosis, psoriasis, Crohn's disease, and type 1 diabetes. Despite their diverse symptoms, autoimmune diseases share several common features, including chronic inflammation, tissue damage, and a range of debilitating symptoms that can impact every aspect of a person's life. One of the most challenging aspects of autoimmune diseases is that they are difficult to diagnose.

They often share symptoms with other conditions, making it difficult for doctors to pinpoint the underlying cause of the symptoms. This can lead to long delays in getting a proper diagnosis and treatment, which can exacerbate the symptoms and make it more difficult to manage the disease.

The first step in understanding autoimmune diseases is to understand the role of the immune system. The immune system is responsible for defending the body against infections, diseases, and foreign invaders. It works by identifying and targeting invading pathogens and neutralizing them before they can cause harm.

In a healthy immune system, the immune cells are able to distinguish between healthy cells and invading pathogens. However, in autoimmune diseases, the immune system becomes confused and starts attacking healthy cells and tissues, leading to chronic inflammation and tissue damage.

The exact causes of autoimmune diseases are not well understood, but several factors have been identified as contributing to their development. These include genetics, environmental factors, and lifestyle factors.

Genetics play a significant role in the development of autoimmune diseases. Family history is often a risk factor for autoimmune diseases, and researchers have identified several genes that may increase a person's risk for autoimmune diseases. However, genetics are not the only factor involved. Environmental factors and lifestyle factors can also play a role in the development of autoimmune diseases.

Environmental factors, such as exposure to toxins, pollutants, and viruses, have been linked to the development of autoimmune diseases. For example, some studies have found that exposure to certain chemicals and pollutants can increase a person's risk for autoimmune diseases.

Lifestyle factors, such as diet, stress, and physical activity, can also play a role in the development of autoimmune diseases. For example, research has found that a diet high in processed foods, sugar, and unhealthy fats can increase inflammation and contribute to the development of autoimmune diseases. Stress can also trigger autoimmune diseases, as it can suppress the immune system and increase inflammation.

Despite the complex and often unknown causes of autoimmune diseases, there are several treatments and lifestyle changes that can help prevent and manage autoimmune diseases. One of the most important is to focus on a healthy diet, including plenty of fruits, vegetables, lean protein, and healthy fats. In addition, stress management techniques, such as exercise, meditation, and deep breathing, can help reduce stress and prevent autoimmune diseases.

Another important aspect of managing autoimmune diseases is to work with a doctor to develop a comprehensive treatment plan. This may include medications, supplements, and lifestyle changes, such as changes to diet and exercise habits.

There is still much to learn about autoimmune diseases, but with the right support and care, people with autoimmune diseases can live healthy and fulfilling lives. Whether it's through lifestyle changes, medication, or a combination of treatments, it is possible to manage autoimmune diseases and reduce their impact on daily life.

The Impact of Autoimmune Diseases on Daily Life

Autoimmune diseases can have a profound impact on daily life, affecting a person's physical, mental, and emotional well-being. These conditions can be painful, debilitating, and can cause a wide range of symptoms, including fatigue, pain, inflammation, and cognitive difficulties.

Physical Impact

One of the most significant impacts of autoimmune diseases is on physical health. People with autoimmune diseases often experience chronic pain and inflammation, which can make it difficult to perform everyday tasks and activities. In some cases, autoimmune diseases can cause permanent joint damage or other physical disabilities, leading to limitations in mobility and independence.

In addition, autoimmune diseases can cause fatigue, making it difficult for people to carry out their daily activities. This can be particularly challenging for people who are employed, as fatigue can make it difficult to concentrate, work effectively, and be productive. People with autoimmune diseases may also experience a range of physical symptoms, such as headaches, muscle weakness, and skin rashes, which can further impact their physical well-being.

Mental Impact

Autoimmune diseases can also have a profound impact on mental health. People with autoimmune diseases often experience feelings of hopelessness, depression, and anxiety. The chronic pain and discomfort caused by autoimmune diseases can make it difficult to enjoy life and participate in daily activities, leading to feelings of isolation and loneliness.

The mental health impact of autoimmune diseases is compounded by the challenges of receiving a proper diagnosis. The diagnostic process for autoimmune diseases can be long and difficult, and many people are misdiagnosed or receive a delayed diagnosis. This can cause feelings of frustration, anger, and confusion, and can further impact mental health.

Emotional Impact

The emotional impact of autoimmune diseases is often underestimated, but it can be just as significant as the physical and mental impacts. People with autoimmune diseases often experience feelings of sadness, frustration, and anger. They may also feel that they are not in control of their own bodies, leading to feelings of hopelessness and despair.

The emotional impact of autoimmune diseases can also affect relationships. People with autoimmune diseases may struggle with intimacy, as pain and discomfort can make it difficult to engage in physical activities. This can lead to feelings of isolation and loneliness, further exacerbating the emotional impact of autoimmune diseases.

Impact on Work and Career

Autoimmune diseases can also have a significant impact on work and career. People with autoimmune diseases may struggle with work-related tasks, such as completing projects, attending meetings, and working long hours. In some cases, autoimmune diseases may result in permanent physical limitations, such as joint damage, which can make it difficult or impossible to continue working.

The impact of autoimmune diseases on work and career can also be compounded by the need for frequent doctor visits and medical appointments. This can lead to missed work days and decreased productivity, making it difficult for people with autoimmune diseases to advance in their careers or maintain their current employment.

Managing the Impact of Autoimmune Diseases

Despite the significant impact of autoimmune diseases on daily life, there are several strategies and treatments that can help manage the impact of these conditions. Some of the most effective strategies include:

Healthy Lifestyle Changes: Maintaining a healthy diet, engaging in regular exercise, and managing stress can help manage the impact of autoimmune diseases. Eating a balanced diet that is rich in anti-inflammatory foods and low in processed foods and sugar can help reduce inflammation and support overall health. Regular exercise can also help improve physical function, reduce pain and fatigue, and improve mental health.

Medications: There are a range of medications that can help manage the symptoms of autoimmune diseases. Anti-inflammatory drugs, such as nonsteroidal anti-inflammatory drugs (NSAIDs), can help reduce pain and inflammation. Corticosteroids can help control inflammation, while immunosuppressant can help control the immune system's overactive response.

Therapies: Therapies such as physical therapy, occupational therapy, and cognitive behavioral therapy can help manage the impact of autoimmune diseases on daily life. Physical therapy can help improve mobility and physical function, while occupational therapy can help with daily activities and work-related tasks. Cognitive behavioral therapy can help manage the emotional impact of autoimmune diseases, and can help with feelings of depression, anxiety, and hopelessness.

Support: Support from family, friends, and support groups can help manage the impact of autoimmune diseases. Talking to others who are going through similar experiences can help reduce feelings of isolation and provide a sense of community.

The Need for a New Approach to Autoimmune Diseases

Autoimmune diseases are a growing problem, affecting millions of people around the world. Despite their prevalence, there is currently no cure for autoimmune diseases, and traditional treatments are often ineffective at addressing the root causes of these conditions. This has led to a growing need for a new approach to autoimmune diseases, one that goes beyond merely managing symptoms and instead addresses the underlying causes of these conditions.

The Limitations of Current Approaches

The current approach to autoimmune diseases is focused on managing symptoms, rather than addressing the root causes of these conditions. This approach typically involves the use of anti-inflammatory drugs, corticosteroids, and immunosuppressant to control inflammation and the immune system's overactive response.

While these medications can help manage symptoms, they do not address the underlying causes of autoimmune diseases and can have serious side effects, including increased risk of infection and long-term damage to organs and tissues.

In addition, current approaches to autoimmune diseases do not take into account the role of lifestyle factors, such as diet, stress, and environmental toxins, in the development and progression of these conditions. As a result, many people with autoimmune diseases are left with limited options for managing their symptoms and improving their health.

The Need for a New Approach

Given the limitations of current approaches to autoimmune diseases, there is a growing need for a new approach that addresses the underlying causes of these conditions and provides a more holistic and comprehensive approach to treatment. This new approach should include:

Addressing the Root Causes: A new approach to autoimmune diseases should focus on addressing the root causes of these conditions, including dietary and lifestyle factors, environmental toxins, and imbalances in the gut microbiome. By addressing the underlying causes of autoimmune diseases, we can help prevent the development of these conditions and reduce the need for medication.

Holistic Approach: A new approach to autoimmune diseases should be holistic, taking into account the interrelated physical, mental, and emotional aspects of these conditions. This includes addressing not just the physical symptoms, but also the emotional and psychological impact of autoimmune diseases on daily life.

Emphasizing Lifestyle Changes: A new approach to autoimmune diseases should emphasize the role of lifestyle changes, including diet and exercise, in the management and prevention of these conditions. By incorporating healthy lifestyle habits, we can help reduce the risk of developing autoimmune diseases and support overall health and well-being.

Integrating Complementary and Alternative Medicine: A new approach to autoimmune diseases should incorporate complementary and alternative medicine, including acupuncture, herbal medicine, and mindfulness-based therapies, as part of a comprehensive treatment plan. These therapies can help manage symptoms, improve overall health, and reduce the need for medication.

The Benefits of a New Approach

A new approach to autoimmune diseases has the potential to provide significant benefits, including:

Improved Outcomes: By addressing the root causes of autoimmune diseases, a new approach has the potential to improve outcomes and provide more effective treatment. This can result in fewer symptoms, reduced pain and discomfort, and improved quality of life.

Reduced Need for Medication: By emphasizing lifestyle changes and incorporating complementary and alternative medicine, a new approach has the potential to reduce the need for medication and its associated side effects.

Improved Mental Health: A new approach that takes into account the interrelated physical, mental, and emotional aspects of autoimmune diseases has the potential to improve mental health and reduce the emotional impact of these conditions.

Increased Awareness: By promoting a more comprehensive and holistic approach to autoimmune diseases, we can increase awareness and understanding of these conditions and help reduce the stigma associated with these conditions.

Chapter 1: The Root Causes of Autoimmune Diseases

The Role of Genetics in Autoimmune Diseases

Autoimmune diseases are a group of chronic conditions in which the body's immune system mistakenly attacks its own tissues and organs. These diseases can affect various parts of the body, including the skin, joints, bones, muscles, and internal organs. Some of the most common autoimmune diseases include rheumatoid arthritis, lupus, multiple sclerosis, and type 1 diabetes.

The exact cause of autoimmune diseases is not known, but it is believed that a combination of genetic, environmental, and lifestyle factors plays a role in the development of these conditions. In this article, we will focus on the role of genetics in autoimmune diseases.

What is Genetics?

Genetics is the study of heredity and the variation of inherited traits. Our genes are the blueprints for the physical and behavioral traits that we inherit from our parents. They are made up of DNA, a chemical code that provides instructions for the development and function of our bodies.

How do Genetics play a role in Autoimmune Diseases?

The role of genetics in autoimmune diseases is complex and multi-faceted. There is no single gene that causes autoimmune diseases, and it is believed that a combination of genetic and environmental factors contributes to their development.

Studies have shown that certain genetic variations are associated with an increased risk of developing autoimmune diseases. These variations are thought to influence the immune system and increase the likelihood of it attacking the body's own tissues and organs.

For example, certain genetic variations have been linked to rheumatoid arthritis, a chronic autoimmune disease that affects the joints. These variations are thought to increase the risk of developing the disease by altering the immune system's response to certain triggers, such as infections or stress.

Similarly, genetic variations have also been linked to other autoimmune diseases, including lupus, multiple sclerosis, and type 1 diabetes. In these diseases, the genetic variations are thought to increase the risk of developing the disease by altering the immune system's response to certain triggers.

Inheritance of Autoimmune Diseases

Autoimmune diseases often run in families, suggesting that there is a genetic component to their development. However, it is important to note that genetics alone do not determine whether or not someone will develop an autoimmune disease.

In many cases, autoimmune diseases are thought to be the result of complex interactions between genetic and environmental factors. For example, a person with a genetic predisposition to a certain autoimmune disease may only develop the disease if they are exposed to certain environmental triggers, such as infections or stress.

This is why some family members with the same genetic variations may not develop the same autoimmune diseases. It is also why some people without a family history of autoimmune diseases may still develop the conditions.

The Impact of Environmental Factors

Environmental factors play a significant role in the development and progression of autoimmune diseases. Autoimmune diseases are a group of conditions in which the immune system mistakenly attacks healthy tissues and organs, causing inflammation, pain, and other symptoms. The exact causes of autoimmune diseases are not well understood, but environmental factors are believed to be a major contributor.

Autoimmune diseases are becoming more common in modern societies, with increasing rates of diagnosis in both industrialized and developing countries.

This suggests that environmental factors are playing a major role in their development and progression. There are several environmental factors that have been identified as contributing to the development of autoimmune diseases, including exposure to toxins and pollutants, dietary changes, and changes in lifestyle and stress levels.

Exposure to Toxins and Pollutants

One of the most significant environmental factors that has been linked to the development of autoimmune diseases is exposure to toxins and pollutants. Toxins and pollutants can come from a variety of sources, including industrial and agricultural processes, household cleaning products, and air and water pollution. Many of these toxins and pollutants are known to disrupt the immune system, causing it to become overactive and attack healthy tissues and organs.

For example, exposure to heavy metals such as lead and mercury has been linked to an increased risk of autoimmune diseases. Heavy metals can interfere with the normal functioning of the immune system, causing it to become overactive and attack healthy tissues. This can lead to inflammation, pain, and other symptoms associated with autoimmune diseases.

Similarly, exposure to pesticides and other chemicals has been linked to an increased risk of autoimmune diseases. Pesticides can disrupt the normal functioning of the immune system, causing it to become overactive and attack healthy tissues. This can result in autoimmune diseases such as rheumatoid arthritis, lupus, and others.

Dietary Changes

Dietary changes have also been linked to the development of autoimmune diseases. A diet high in processed foods, sugar, and unhealthy fats can increase inflammation in the body, which can contribute to the development of autoimmune diseases. In contrast, a diet that is rich in nutrients and anti-inflammatory foods has been shown to reduce the risk of autoimmune diseases.

For example, a diet that is high in processed foods, sugar, and unhealthy fats can lead to an imbalance in gut bacteria, which has been linked to an increased risk of autoimmune diseases. An imbalance in gut bacteria can cause inflammation in the gut, which can disrupt the normal functioning of the immune system and increase the risk of autoimmune diseases.

In contrast, a diet that is rich in nutrient-dense foods, such as fruits, vegetables, and whole grains, can help to reduce inflammation in the body. This can reduce the risk of autoimmune diseases and improve overall health. Additionally, consuming probiotics, such as fermented foods and drinks, can help to restore balance to the gut microbiome, reducing inflammation and reducing the risk of autoimmune diseases.

Lifestyle and Stress Changes

Lifestyle and stress changes are also believed to contribute to the development of autoimmune diseases. A sedentary lifestyle, combined with high levels of stress, can increase inflammation in the body, contributing to the development of autoimmune diseases.

For example, a sedentary lifestyle can increase oxidative stress in the body, which can contribute to inflammation and the development of autoimmune diseases. Similarly, high levels of stress can disrupt the normal functioning of the immune system, causing it to become overactive and attack healthy tissues. This can lead to autoimmune diseases such as lupus, rheumatoid arthritis, and others.

In contrast, a healthy lifestyle, which includes regular physical activity, stress management techniques, and a balanced diet, can reduce inflammation in the body and reduce the risk of autoimmune diseases.

The Role of Gut Health

The role of gut health has become increasingly recognized in recent years, with more and more research pointing to its importance in overall health and well-being. The gut, also known as the digestive system, is a complex network of organs that are responsible for the processing of food, the extraction of nutrients, and the elimination of waste.

The gut also plays a crucial role in the health of the immune system, as well as the production of hormones and neurotransmitters that affect our mood and mental state. In this article, we will explore the role of gut health in detail, including its impact on overall health, the factors that contribute to poor gut health, and the ways in which it can be improved.

The gut is home to a diverse community of microorganisms, known as the gut microbiome. This microbiome plays a critical role in maintaining gut health and overall well-being. The gut microbiome acts as a barrier, preventing harmful pathogens from entering the body, and also helps to break down food and extract nutrients.

A healthy gut microbiome is essential for maintaining a strong immune system, as it helps to prevent infections and other illnesses. In addition, the gut microbiome helps to regulate the production of hormones and neurotransmitters, which play a role in mood and mental health.

However, a number of factors can contribute to poor gut health and disrupt the balance of the gut microbiome. These include a diet high in processed foods, antibiotics, and other medications, chronic stress, and a sedentary lifestyle. When the balance of the gut microbiome is disrupted, harmful bacteria can overgrow, leading to symptoms such as bloating, gas, diarrhea, and constipation. In addition, poor gut health can lead to an increased risk of chronic diseases, including autoimmune disorders, cardiovascular disease, and type 2 diabetes.

One of the key ways to improve gut health is through diet. A diet that is high in fiber, fermented foods, and probiotics can help to support a healthy gut microbiome. Fiber is essential for feeding the beneficial bacteria in the gut, while fermented foods and probiotics can help to repopulate the gut with beneficial bacteria.

Additionally, reducing the consumption of processed foods, sugar, and unhealthy fats can help to improve gut health by reducing inflammation and promoting the growth of beneficial bacteria.

In addition to diet, lifestyle changes can also play a role in improving gut health. Regular physical activity can help to reduce stress and promote gut health, as well as improve overall health.

Stress reduction techniques, such as mindfulness, yoga, and deep breathing, can also be helpful in reducing stress and promoting gut health. Additionally, getting adequate sleep and managing stress levels can help to improve gut health and reduce the risk of chronic diseases.

Finally, supplementing with probiotics and prebiotics can also help to improve gut health. Probiotics are live bacteria and yeast that are beneficial for the gut, while prebiotics are fibers that feed the beneficial bacteria in the gut. These supplements can help to repopulate the gut with beneficial bacteria, reduce inflammation, and improve gut health.

The Impact of Stress and Lifestyle Factors

Stress and lifestyle factors have a profound impact on our overall health and well-being. In recent years, a growing body of research has linked these factors to a range of health problems, including autoimmune diseases.

Autoimmune diseases are a group of disorders in which the immune system attacks the body's own tissues and organs, leading to chronic inflammation and tissue damage. The exact causes of autoimmune diseases are still not fully understood, but it is clear that stress and lifestyle factors play a key role in their development and progression.

What is stress?

Stress is a natural response to perceived threats, and it is a normal part of life. When we experience stress, our bodies release hormones such as cortisol and adrenaline, which prepare us to take action. In the short term, stress can be beneficial, as it can help us respond to challenges and situations that require us to be alert and focused.

However, when stress becomes chronic, it can have a profound impact on our health and well-being. Chronic stress has been linked to a wide range of health problems, including cardiovascular disease, depression, anxiety, and autoimmune diseases.

What are lifestyle factors?

Lifestyle factors are a range of habits, behaviors, and environmental factors that impact our health and well-being. Some common lifestyle factors that have been linked to autoimmune diseases include diet, physical activity levels, exposure to toxins, and sleep patterns. While many of these factors are under our control, they can be influenced by external factors such as our social and economic circumstances, as well as our environment and personal relationships.

The impact of stress on autoimmune diseases

One of the key ways in which stress affects autoimmune diseases is by compromising the function of the immune system. When we experience stress, our bodies release hormones such as cortisol and adrenaline, which can have a negative impact on the immune system.

For example, cortisol can suppress the function of certain cells in the immune system, reducing their ability to fight off infections and respond to foreign invaders. This can leave us vulnerable to a range of health problems, including autoimmune diseases.

In addition to compromising the function of the immune system, stress has been linked to a range of other factors that can contribute to the development and progression of autoimmune diseases. For example, stress can affect our gut health, leading to changes in the balance of bacteria in our gut microbiome.

These changes can lead to gut permeability, a condition in which harmful bacteria and toxins enter the bloodstream and trigger an immune response. This immune response can then contribute to the development and progression of autoimmune diseases.

Stress can also affect our diet and lifestyle habits, leading us to make unhealthy choices that can further contribute to the development of autoimmune diseases. For example, stress can lead to overeating, increased alcohol consumption, and reduced physical activity levels, all of which can have a negative impact on our health.

The impact of lifestyle factors on autoimmune diseases

Lifestyle factors also play a key role in the development and progression of autoimmune diseases. Diet, in particular, has been linked to a range of autoimmune diseases, including rheumatoid arthritis, lupus, and multiple sclerosis.

Certain foods, such as gluten and dairy, have been shown to trigger an immune response in some individuals, leading to inflammation and tissue damage. On the other hand, a diet rich in anti-inflammatory foods, such as fruits, vegetables, and healthy fats, can help to reduce inflammation and support the immune system.

Physical activity levels have also been linked to autoimmune diseases. Regular exercise has been shown to have a positive impact on the immune system, reducing inflammation and improving overall health.

In contrast, a sedentary lifestyle has been linked to a range of health problems, including an increased risk of developing autoimmune diseases. Inactivity has also been linked to a decline in gut health, which can further contribute to the development and progression of autoimmune diseases.

Exposure to toxins can also play a role in the development of autoimmune diseases. Toxins, such as heavy metals and chemicals, can trigger an immune response and lead to chronic inflammation. This can be particularly harmful to individuals who are already prone to autoimmune diseases.

Sleep patterns are another important factor in the development of autoimmune diseases. Sleep plays a crucial role in regulating the immune system, and a lack of sleep has been linked to a range of health problems, including autoimmune diseases. When we sleep, our bodies produce cytokines, which are chemical signals that help to regulate the immune system. Lack of sleep can disrupt this process, leading to changes in the balance of cytokines and an increased risk of developing autoimmune diseases.

Chapter 2: The Autoimmune Solution

The Four-Step Program for Preventing and Reversing Autoimmune Diseases

Autoimmune diseases are a growing problem in the modern world, affecting millions of people worldwide. These diseases are characterized by the body's immune system attacking healthy tissues, resulting in a range of symptoms such as joint pain, fatigue, and digestive problems.

The conventional approach to autoimmune diseases typically involves taking medication to suppress the immune system, but this approach often comes with unwanted side effects and does not address the root causes of autoimmune diseases.

The good news is that there is a revolutionary approach to preventing and reversing autoimmune diseases, and it is called the four-step program. This program is designed to address the root causes of autoimmune diseases and support the body's natural healing mechanisms, resulting in better health outcomes for people with autoimmune diseases. In this article, we will explore the four-step program in detail and provide insights into how it can be used to prevent and reverse autoimmune diseases.

Step 1: Remove

The first step in the four-step program for preventing and reversing autoimmune diseases is to remove autoimmune triggers. Autoimmune triggers are substances or factors that cause the immune system to attack healthy tissues, leading to autoimmune diseases. Common autoimmune triggers include gluten, dairy, and soy, but there are many other triggers that can be specific to each individual.

To identify and remove autoimmune triggers, it is important to undergo a food elimination diet. This involves removing common allergens and irritants from the diet and gradually reintroducing them to determine which foods trigger an autoimmune response. Once the autoimmune triggers have been identified, they should be avoided to prevent further immune system damage.

In addition to food elimination, it is also important to avoid processed foods and chemicals that can disrupt the gut microbiome and trigger an autoimmune response. These chemicals are often found in household and personal care products, so it is essential to use natural alternatives and read labels carefully.

Step 2: Replace

The second step in the four-step program for preventing and reversing autoimmune diseases is to replace nutrient-deficient foods with nutrient-dense foods. Autoimmune diseases are often caused by nutrient deficiencies, particularly in vitamins and minerals such as vitamin D, zinc, and magnesium. Replacing nutrient-deficient foods with nutrient-dense foods can help to support the immune system and prevent autoimmune diseases.

Examples of nutrient-dense foods include leafy greens, nuts, seeds, and high-quality proteins such as grass-fed beef, wild-caught fish, and free-range eggs. It is also important to incorporate healthy fats into the diet, as they are essential for optimal immune function. Examples of healthy fats include avocado, olive oil, and coconut oil.

In addition to a nutrient-dense diet, it is also important to take supplements and vitamins to support the immune system. Vitamin D, magnesium, and zinc are particularly important for preventing and reversing autoimmune diseases. It is also essential to include probiotics and fermented foods in the diet to support gut health and improve the gut microbiome.

Step 3: Reinoculate

The third step in the four-step program for preventing and reversing autoimmune diseases is to reinoculate the gut with beneficial bacteria. The gut microbiome is a critical component of the immune system, and imbalances in the gut microbiome can trigger an autoimmune response. To support the gut microbiome and prevent autoimmune diseases, it is important to reinoculate the gut with beneficial bacteria through probiotics and fermented foods.

Probiotics are live microorganisms that are taken as a supplement or found in fermented foods such as kimchi, kefir, and sauerkraut. Probiotics help to balance the gut microbiome and improve gut health, resulting in better immune function and a reduced risk of autoimmune diseases.

In addition to probiotics, prebiotics are also important for reinforcing the gut microbiome. Prebiotics are indigestible fibers that feed the beneficial bacteria in the gut, allowing them to thrive and promote healthy gut function. Foods high in prebiotics include garlic, onions, leeks, and asparagus.

Step 4: Repair

The final step in the four-step program for preventing and reversing autoimmune diseases is to repair the gut lining. The gut lining is a critical component of the immune system, as it serves as a barrier to prevent harmful substances from entering the body.

In people with autoimmune diseases, the gut lining is often damaged, allowing harmful substances to enter the body and trigger an autoimmune response.

To repair the gut lining, it is essential to address gut inflammation and improve gut health. This can be done through a nutrient-dense diet, probiotics and prebiotics, and supplements such as L-glutamine and aloe Vera. It is also important to avoid gut irritants, such as processed foods and chemicals, to reduce further gut damage.

The Importance of Nutrition and Supplementation

Nutrition and supplementation play a crucial role in our overall health and well-being. In the context of autoimmune diseases, these two factors are especially important in preventing and reversing the symptoms and consequences of these chronic conditions.

Autoimmune diseases are a group of conditions in which the immune system mistakenly attacks the body's own cells, leading to inflammation and damage to various tissues and organs. The causes of autoimmune diseases are complex and multifactorial, but nutrition and supplementation can play a key role in mitigating the effects of these diseases. In this article, we will discuss the importance of nutrition and supplementation in the context of autoimmune diseases and provide some practical advice and recommendations for those affected by these conditions.

The Importance of Nutrition in Autoimmune Diseases

Nutrition is a critical factor in maintaining a healthy immune system and preventing autoimmune diseases. The foods we eat can directly impact the function and balance of our immune system, as well as the health and function of the gut, which is considered the "command center" of the immune system.

The gut is lined with a barrier of cells and mucus that prevents harmful substances from entering the bloodstream and triggering an immune response. If this barrier is damaged, harmful substances can enter the bloodstream and trigger an autoimmune response.

In order to maintain a healthy gut and immune system, it is important to eat a diet that is high in nutrients and low in inflammatory foods. A diet that is rich in fresh fruits and vegetables, healthy fats, lean proteins, and whole grains can help support the health of the gut and immune system.

In contrast, a diet that is high in processed foods, refined sugars, and unhealthy fats can damage the gut barrier and trigger an autoimmune response.

Some specific foods and nutrients that are important for the health of the gut and immune system include:

Probiotics: These are beneficial bacteria that live in the gut and play a key role in maintaining gut health. Probiotics can be found in fermented foods such as yogurt, kefir, and sauerkraut.

Fiber: Fiber is essential for maintaining the health of the gut by promoting regular bowel movements and supporting the growth of beneficial bacteria.

Omega-3 fatty acids: These healthy fats have anti-inflammatory effects and can help reduce the risk of autoimmune diseases. Omega-3 fatty acids can be found in fatty fish, nuts, and seeds.

Vitamins and minerals: Vitamins and minerals are essential for the proper functioning of the immune system and the maintenance of a healthy gut. Some of the most important vitamins and minerals for autoimmune diseases include vitamin D, vitamin B12, and iron.

The Importance of Supplementation in Autoimmune Diseases

In addition to a healthy diet, supplementation can also play a key role in preventing and reversing autoimmune diseases. Some of the most important supplements for autoimmune diseases include:

Probiotics: Probiotics are beneficial bacteria that can help restore the balance of the gut microbiome and support the health of the gut and immune system.

Omega-3 fatty acids: Omega-3 fatty acids can help reduce inflammation and support the health of the immune system.

Vitamin D: Vitamin D is important for the proper functioning of the immune system and can help reduce the risk of autoimmune diseases.

Vitamin B12: Vitamin B12 is important for the health of the nervous system and the production of red blood cells.

Iron: Iron is essential for the proper functioning of the immune system and the maintenance of a healthy gut.

In addition to these specific supplements, it is also important to take a multivitamin that contains a wide range of essential vitamins and minerals. This can help ensure that you are getting all of the nutrients you need to support the health of your immune system and reduce the risk of autoimmune diseases.

However, it is important to keep in mind that not all supplements are created equal, and it is important to choose high-quality supplements that are manufactured by reputable companies. It is also important to talk to your doctor before starting any new supplement regimen, as some supplements can interact with medications or other health conditions.

Another important aspect of supplementation for autoimmune diseases is the use of immune-modulating supplements. These supplements can help regulate the immune system and reduce the risk of autoimmune diseases. Some of the most commonly used immune-modulating supplements include:

Curcumin: This is the active ingredient in turmeric and has potent anti-inflammatory effects.

Ginger: Ginger has anti-inflammatory and antioxidant effects and can help reduce the risk of autoimmune diseases.

Resveratrol: This is a compound found in red wine and has anti-inflammatory effects.

Quercetin: This is a natural antioxidant found in many fruits and vegetables and has anti-inflammatory effects.

Understanding the Connection between the Gut and the Immune System

The human body is a complex system with many interconnected parts. The gut and the immune system are two important systems that have a close relationship with each other. The gut is responsible for processing the food we eat and absorbing nutrients, while the immune system protects us from disease and infection.

The gut and the immune system are connected in several ways, and a disrupted gut microbiome can lead to a weakened immune system, while a weakened immune system can lead to gut problems. Understanding the connection between the gut and the immune system is crucial for maintaining good health and preventing autoimmune diseases.

The Gut Microbiome:

The gut microbiome refers to the collection of microbes, including bacteria, viruses, and fungi, that live in our gut. It is estimated that there are over 100 trillion microbes in our gut, which outnumber our own cells by 10 to 1.

These microbes play a crucial role in our health by regulating digestion, absorption of nutrients, and the production of hormones. They also help to maintain a healthy immune system by preventing the growth of harmful bacteria and promoting the growth of beneficial bacteria.

The gut microbiome is a complex and dynamic system that is influenced by many factors, including diet, lifestyle, and the use of antibiotics. An imbalanced gut microbiome can lead to gut problems, such as diarrhea, constipation, and irritable bowel syndrome. It can also lead to a weakened immune system and increase the risk of autoimmune diseases.

The Immune System:

The immune system is a complex network of cells and tissues that protect the body from disease and infection. The immune system is divided into two main branches: the innate immune system and the adaptive immune system.

The innate immune system is the first line of defense against infection and includes physical barriers such as the skin, mucous membranes, and gut bacteria. The adaptive immune system is responsible for recognizing and eliminating specific pathogens and includes T and B cells.

The gut and the immune system interact with each other in several ways. The gut microbiome helps to train the immune system by exposing it to a variety of microbes and promoting the development of immune cells.

The gut also contains immune cells, such as T cells and B cells, that help to maintain a healthy immune system. In addition, the gut produces cytokines and other signaling molecules that help to regulate the immune system.

The Connection between the Gut and the Immune System:

The connection between the gut and the immune system is complex and bidirectional. A disrupted gut microbiome can lead to a weakened immune system, while a weakened immune system can lead to gut problems. Some of the ways in which the gut and the immune system interact include:

Gut Permeability: The gut is lined with a thin layer of cells called the epithelial barrier. This barrier helps to keep harmful substances and pathogens out of the bloodstream and maintain a healthy gut microbiome. However, a disrupted gut microbiome can lead to an increase in gut permeability, allowing harmful substances and pathogens to leak into the bloodstream and trigger an immune response. This can lead to a weakened immune system and increase the risk of autoimmune diseases.

Immune Cells in the Gut: The gut is home to a variety of immune cells, including T cells, B cells, and innate immune cells. These immune cells help to maintain a healthy gut microbiome by regulating the growth of harmful bacteria and promoting the growth of beneficial bacteria. In addition, they help to prevent infections and inflammation. A disrupted gut microbiome can lead to a decrease in immune cells in the gut, resulting in a weakened immune system and increased risk of autoimmune diseases.

Cytokines and Signaling Molecules: The gut produces a variety of cytokines and signaling molecules that help to regulate the immune system. These signaling molecules help to regulate the activity of immune cells, including T and B cells, and can either stimulate or suppress the immune response.

In a healthy gut microbiome, the production of cytokines and signaling molecules is balanced, promoting a strong immune response. However, in a disrupted gut microbiome, an imbalance in the production of these signaling molecules can result in a weakened immune system and increase the risk of autoimmune diseases.

Gut-Liver Axis: The gut and the liver also have a close connection known as the gut-liver axis. The liver helps to filter toxins and waste products from the bloodstream, and a healthy gut microbiome is important for maintaining liver function. A disrupted gut microbiome can lead to an increase in gut permeability, allowing harmful substances and toxins to enter the bloodstream and cause liver damage. This can result in a weakened immune system and increase the risk of autoimmune diseases.

Diet and Lifestyle: Diet and lifestyle play a significant role in the connection between the gut and the immune system. A diet high in processed foods, sugar, and unhealthy fats can disrupt the gut microbiome, leading to a weakened immune system and increased risk of autoimmune diseases. On the other hand, a diet high in fiber, fruits, and vegetables can help to promote a healthy gut microbiome and support a strong immune system. Additionally, lifestyle factors such as stress, lack of sleep, and physical inactivity can also disrupt the gut microbiome and weaken the immune system.

Chapter 3: Step 1: Remove

Identifying and Removing Autoimmune Triggers

Identifying and removing autoimmune triggers is a critical step in the autoimmune solution and a key factor in preventing and reversing autoimmune diseases. Autoimmune diseases are a group of conditions where the immune system mistakenly attacks healthy cells and tissues, leading to chronic inflammation and the development of various diseases such as rheumatoid arthritis, lupus, and multiple sclerosis.

The causes of autoimmune diseases are complex and multifactorial, but identifying and removing triggers can play a crucial role in reducing symptoms and improving overall health.

What are autoimmune triggers?

Autoimmune triggers are factors that trigger an immune response and contribute to the development and progression of autoimmune diseases. They can be a variety of things such as food allergens, environmental toxins, infections, stress, and medications. Some of the most common autoimmune triggers include gluten, dairy, soy, corn, eggs, and nuts. It is important to note that not all triggers will be the same for everyone, and each individual's triggers will vary based on their genetics, environment, and lifestyle.

How to identify autoimmune triggers?

The first step in identifying autoimmune triggers is to keep a detailed food and symptom diary. This will allow you to see any correlations between the foods you eat and the symptoms you experience. It is important to note that symptoms may not appear immediately after eating a trigger food, and it can take several days for symptoms to manifest. Once you have identified potential trigger foods, you can eliminate them from your diet for several weeks and observe any changes in symptoms. If symptoms improve, you can then gradually reintroduce the food and see if symptoms return.

Another way to identify autoimmune triggers is through food intolerance testing. This can be done through a blood test, skin prick test, or elimination diet. These tests will identify any food sensitivities that may be contributing to autoimmune symptoms.

Environmental toxins and infections can also play a role in triggering autoimmune symptoms. It is important to reduce your exposure to these triggers by avoiding exposure to chemicals, such as pesticides and cleaning products, and practicing good hygiene to reduce the risk of infections. Stress can also be a trigger for autoimmune diseases, and it is important to manage stress through relaxation techniques, such as meditation and yoga, and regular exercise.

Medications can also trigger autoimmune symptoms, and it is important to discuss any medications you are taking with your healthcare provider to determine if they may be contributing to your symptoms.

Removing autoimmune triggers

Once you have identified your autoimmune triggers, the next step is to remove them from your diet and lifestyle. This can involve eliminating certain foods, reducing exposure to environmental toxins, and managing stress.

Eliminating trigger foods

Eliminating trigger foods is a crucial step in reducing autoimmune symptoms. It is important to remove all sources of the trigger food, including hidden sources, such as sauces and processed foods. Some individuals may choose to follow a specific diet, such as the autoimmune protocol (AIP) diet, which eliminates certain foods and focuses on nutrient-dense, whole foods.

Reducing exposure to environmental toxins

Reducing exposure to environmental toxins is another important step in removing autoimmune triggers. This can involve using natural cleaning products, reducing exposure to chemicals, such as pesticides, and choosing products made from organic and non-toxic materials.

Managing stress

Stress is a well-known trigger for autoimmune diseases, and it is important to manage stress through relaxation techniques, such as meditation and yoga, and regular exercise. Additionally, it is important to prioritize self-care, such as getting adequate sleep and maintaining a healthy work-life balance.

The role of gut healing in removing autoimmune triggers

Gut health is a critical factor in autoimmune diseases, and it is crucial to heal the gut to reduce autoimmune symptoms. The gut is home to a large number of beneficial bacteria, also known as the gut microbiome, which play a crucial role in regulating the immune system and reducing inflammation. When the gut microbiome is disrupted, it can lead to an overactive immune response and the development of autoimmune diseases.

To heal the gut, it is important to follow an anti-inflammatory diet, such as the autoimmune protocol diet, which eliminates trigger foods and focuses on nutrient-dense, whole foods. It is also important to incorporate probiotics and fermented foods into your diet, such as kefir, sauerkraut, and kimchi, to improve gut health and reduce inflammation. Additionally, it is important to avoid antibiotics, which can disrupt the gut microbiome, and to manage stress, which can also negatively impact gut health.

How to Eliminate Common Allergens and Irritants

Allergens and irritants are common triggers for autoimmune diseases and other health conditions. These triggers can cause inflammation and damage to the gut lining, leading to a variety of symptoms and exacerbating autoimmune diseases. Therefore, eliminating common allergens and irritants from your diet and environment is an important step in preventing and reversing autoimmune diseases. In this article, we will discuss how to identify common allergens and irritants and provide tips for removing them from your life.

Identifying Common Allergens and Irritants:

The first step in eliminating allergens and irritants is to identify them. This can be done through a variety of methods, including food elimination diets, skin prick tests, and blood tests. A food elimination diet involves removing common allergens from your diet and gradually reintroducing them to see if they cause symptoms.

Skin prick tests and blood tests can help identify specific allergens that may be triggering your symptoms.

Common allergens and irritants include:

Gluten: Gluten is a protein found in wheat, barley, and rye that can cause an autoimmune reaction in some people with celiac disease or non-celiac gluten sensitivity.

Dairy: Many people are intolerant to lactose, the sugar found in dairy products, or have an allergy to the protein casein.

Soy: Soy is a common allergen that can cause symptoms in people with soy allergies.

Nuts: Nut allergies are common and can cause severe reactions in some people.

Shellfish: Shellfish allergies are common and can cause severe reactions in some people.

Chemicals: Chemical allergens can be found in food, cleaning products, and personal care products.

Common chemical allergens include food additives, artificial sweeteners, and fragrances.

Molds: Mold allergies are common and can cause symptoms such as sneezing, itching, and skin rashes.

Removing Allergens and Irritants from Your Diet:

Once you have identified common allergens and irritants, the next step is to remove them from your diet. This can be challenging, especially if you have a busy lifestyle, but it is important to take the time to make changes to your diet to help prevent and reverse autoimmune diseases.

Gluten: To remove gluten from your diet, avoid foods that contain wheat, barley, and rye, including bread, pasta, and baked goods. Instead, opt for gluten-free grains such as quinoa, brown rice, and millet.

Dairy: To remove dairy from your diet, avoid all dairy products, including milk, cheese, and yogurt. Instead, opt for non-dairy alternatives such as almond milk, coconut yogurt, and nut-based cheeses.

Soy: To remove soy from your diet, avoid foods that contain soy, such as tofu, soy milk, and soy sauce. Instead, opt for soy-free alternatives such as almond milk, coconut yogurt, and nut-based cheeses.

Nuts: To remove nuts from your diet, avoid all nut products, including nut butters, nut milks, and baked goods. Instead, opt for nut-free alternatives such as sunflower seed butter and almond flour.

Shellfish: To remove shellfish from your diet, avoid all shellfish products, including shrimp, crab, and lobster.

Chemicals: To remove chemicals from your diet, avoid processed foods and opt for whole, fresh foods instead. Read labels carefully to avoid foods that contain artificial sweeteners, preservatives, and food dyes.

The Importance of Avoiding Processed Foods and Chemicals

In recent years, there has been a growing awareness of the impact that food and the environment have on our health. One of the biggest contributors to poor health is the consumption of processed foods and chemicals.

These foods and chemicals have been linked to numerous health problems, including autoimmune diseases, chronic inflammation, and even cancer. In this article, we will explore the reasons why it is so important to avoid processed foods and chemicals and what steps you can take to minimize your exposure to them.

Processed Foods

Processed foods are those that have been altered from their natural state in some way. This can include things like adding preservatives, artificial colors and flavors, or using heat or chemical treatments. Processed foods are often high in sugar, salt, and unhealthy fats, and low in essential nutrients. They can also contain harmful additives, such as high fructose corn syrup, monosodium glutamate (MSG), and artificial sweeteners, that can have negative effects on our health.

One of the biggest problems with processed foods is that they are often high in calories and low in nutrients. This can lead to weight gain and other health problems, such as heart disease, high blood pressure, and type 2 diabetes. Processed foods are also often high in unhealthy fats, such as trans fats, which have been linked to numerous health problems, including heart disease, stroke, and cancer.

Another problem with processed foods is that they can be high in chemicals, such as preservatives, artificial colors, and artificial flavors. These chemicals can have a negative impact on our health, and may contribute to chronic inflammation, which has been linked to a number of health problems, including autoimmune diseases and cancer.

Chemicals in Processed Foods

There are many chemicals that are commonly used in processed foods, and some of them have been linked to negative health effects. Some of the most common chemicals include:

Bisphenol-A (BPA) - BPA is a chemical that is used to make plastic containers and cans. It has been linked to numerous health problems, including hormone imbalances, infertility, and cancer.

Phthalates - Phthalates are a group of chemicals that are used to make plastics and other consumer products. They have been linked to numerous health problems, including hormone imbalances, infertility, and cancer.

High Fructose Corn Syrup (HFCS) - HFCS is a sweetener that is commonly used in processed foods, including candy, soda, and other sweets. It has been linked to numerous health problems, including weight gain, type 2 diabetes, and heart disease.

Artificial Sweeteners - Artificial sweeteners are often used in place of sugar in processed foods. They have been linked to numerous health problems, including weight gain, insulin resistance, and cancer.

Monosodium Glutamate (MSG) - MSG is a flavor enhancer that is commonly used in processed foods, including soups, broths, and processed meats. It has been linked to numerous health problems, including headaches, migraines, and heart disease.

Avoiding Processed Foods and Chemicals

The best way to avoid processed foods and chemicals is to eat a diet that is based on whole, unprocessed foods. This means eating plenty of fruits and vegetables, whole grains, lean proteins, and healthy fats. It also means avoiding processed foods and chemicals as much as possible.

Here are some tips for avoiding processed foods and chemicals:

Read food labels carefully. When shopping, take the time to read food labels and look for foods that are made with whole, unprocessed ingredients.

Avoid processed snacks and sweets. Instead, opt for fresh fruit or nuts for a snack.

Cook at home as much as possible. This will allow you to control what ingredients go into your food and avoid processed foods and chemicals.

Use glass or stainless steel containers instead of plastic containers. BPA and phthalates can leach out of plastic containers and into your food.

Choose organic produce whenever possible. Organic produce is grown without the use of harmful pesticides and chemicals.

Avoid artificial sweeteners and choose natural sweeteners instead, such as honey or maple syrup.

Be mindful of what you drink. Avoid soda and other sweetened drinks, which are often high in chemicals and unhealthy sugars. Instead, drink water, herbal teas, and other healthy drinks.

Limit your exposure to environmental chemicals. This includes avoiding products that contain chemicals like phthalates and BPA, and limiting your exposure to pollutants in the air and water.

The Role of Gut Healing Diets in Autoimmune Diseases

One of the most important factors in the development of autoimmune diseases is gut health. The gut is the largest immune organ in the body and is responsible for regulating the immune system and preventing harmful pathogens from entering the body. When the gut is damaged or becomes imbalanced, the immune system can become hyperactive and attack the body's own tissues, leading to autoimmune disease.

To prevent and manage autoimmune diseases, it is essential to heal the gut and restore balance to the gut microbiome. One of the most effective ways to do this is through the use of gut healing diets. Gut healing diets are specialized diets that focus on removing foods that can damage the gut and replacing them with foods that promote gut health.

The most well-known gut healing diet is the autoimmune protocol (AIP), which is designed specifically for people with autoimmune diseases. The AIP diet eliminates foods that are known to cause inflammation and harm the gut, such as gluten, dairy, soy, and refined sugars, and replaces them with nutrient-dense foods such as vegetables, meats, and healthy fats. The AIP diet also emphasizes the consumption of probiotics, fermented foods, and other foods that promote gut health.

Another popular gut healing diet is the low-FODMAP diet, which stands for Fermentable Oligosaccharides, Disaccharides, Monosaccharides, and Polyols. This diet eliminates foods that are high in short-chain carbohydrates that are difficult to digest and can lead to gut inflammation, such as onions, garlic, and wheat. By removing these foods, the low-FODMAP diet helps to reduce gut inflammation and improve gut health.

The gut and psychology syndrome (GAPS) diet is another gut healing diet that focuses on restoring gut health and balancing the gut microbiome. This diet eliminates grains, refined sugars, and processed foods and emphasizes the consumption of nutrient-dense foods such as meats, vegetables, and healthy fats. The GAPS diet also includes the consumption of fermented foods and probiotics to help restore gut health.

In addition to these specific gut healing diets, there are also general dietary principles that are recommended for people with autoimmune diseases. These principles include eating a diet rich in nutrient-dense foods, such as vegetables, meats, and healthy fats, and avoiding processed foods and refined sugars. It is also recommended to consume probiotics and fermented foods to promote gut health and to limit the consumption of gluten, dairy, soy, and other foods that can harm the gut.

The role of gut healing diets in autoimmune diseases is becoming increasingly recognized by the medical community. Many studies have shown that by healing the gut and restoring balance to the gut microbiome, people with autoimmune diseases can reduce inflammation, improve symptoms, and even reverse the progression of the disease.

For example, one study found that people with rheumatoid arthritis who followed a gut healing diet experienced significant improvements in their symptoms, including a reduction in pain and inflammation. Another study found that people with multiple sclerosis who followed a gut healing diet experienced an improvement in their symptoms and a reduction in the progression of the disease.

Chapter 4: Step 2: Replace

The Role of Nutrient-Dense Foods in Autoimmune Disease

While there are many different factors that contribute to the development of autoimmune diseases, one of the most important is diet. In particular, the role of nutrient-dense foods in autoimmune disease cannot be overstated.

Nutrient-dense foods are those that provide a high amount of essential vitamins, minerals, and antioxidants per calorie. These foods are critical for maintaining overall health and reducing the risk of chronic diseases, including autoimmune diseases. In order to understand the role of nutrient-dense foods in autoimmune disease, it is first necessary to understand the impact of diet on the immune system.

The immune system is a complex network of cells and tissues that work together to protect the body from harm. In order for the immune system to function optimally, it needs to be fueled by a balanced and nutritious diet. Nutrient-dense foods provide the necessary vitamins, minerals, and antioxidants to support a healthy immune system.

For example, vitamin C is an antioxidant that has been shown to enhance immune function, while vitamin D plays a critical role in regulating immune responses.

In addition to vitamins and minerals, nutrient-dense foods also contain essential fatty acids, which are critical for maintaining the integrity of the cell membrane. These fatty acids help to protect cells from damage and support the immune system in identifying and attacking foreign invaders. Omega-3 fatty acids, in particular, have been shown to have anti-inflammatory properties and are crucial for reducing the risk of autoimmune diseases.

Nutrient-dense foods are also important for maintaining gut health. The gut is a critical component of the immune system, serving as the first line of defense against harmful pathogens. When the gut is healthy, it is able to identify and eliminate harmful substances before they can reach the rest of the body. However, when the gut is damaged, it becomes permeable, allowing harmful substances to enter the bloodstream and trigger an autoimmune response.

Nutrient-dense foods are critical for repairing and maintaining the gut lining. For example, probiotics are a type of beneficial bacteria that are essential for gut health. Probiotics help to maintain the balance of good and bad bacteria in the gut, which is critical for reducing the risk of autoimmune diseases. In addition, prebiotics are types of fibers that feed the good bacteria in the gut, helping to maintain gut health.

When it comes to autoimmune diseases, the role of nutrient-dense foods cannot be overstated. For example, those with autoimmune diseases such as rheumatoid arthritis, psoriasis, and lupus often have imbalanced gut bacteria and a compromised gut lining. In order to reduce the risk of autoimmune diseases, it is important to consume a diet that is rich in nutrient-dense foods that support gut health.

In addition to reducing the risk of autoimmune diseases, nutrient-dense foods can also help to manage existing autoimmune conditions. For example, a diet rich in nutrient-dense foods has been shown to reduce inflammation, which is a hallmark of autoimmune diseases. Inflammation is the body's natural response to injury or infection, but in autoimmune diseases, it becomes chronic and can lead to tissue damage. By reducing inflammation through a diet rich in nutrient-dense foods, it is possible to manage autoimmune diseases and improve overall health.

There are many different nutrient-dense foods that can be incorporated into a diet to support health and reduce the risk of autoimmune diseases. Some of the most important include:

Leafy greens: Leafy greens, such as spinach, kale, and collard greens, are packed with vitamins, minerals, and antioxidants. These foods are high in vitamin C, which has been shown to enhance immune function, and vitamin K, which is important for maintaining healthy bones. Leafy greens are also rich in folate, which is critical for cell division and growth.

Berries: Berries, such as blueberries, strawberries, and raspberries, are high in antioxidants and anti-inflammatory compounds. These foods are also high in vitamin C, which supports the immune system. Berries are a great source of fiber, which helps to maintain gut health.

Nuts and seeds: Nuts and seeds, such as almonds, walnuts, and chia seeds, are high in essential fatty acids and protein. They are also rich in magnesium, which is important for maintaining healthy bones and reducing inflammation. Nuts and seeds are also a great source of antioxidants, which help to protect cells from damage.

Fermented foods: Fermented foods, such as yogurt, kefir, and sauerkraut, are high in probiotics and prebiotics. These foods help to maintain the balance of good and bad bacteria in the gut, which is critical for reducing the risk of autoimmune diseases. Fermented foods also contain anti-inflammatory compounds that help to reduce inflammation.

Meat and fish: Meat and fish, such as chicken, beef, and salmon, are high in protein and essential fatty acids. These foods are also rich in B vitamins, which are important for energy metabolism and supporting the immune system. Fish, in particular, is a great source of omega-3 fatty acids, which have anti-inflammatory properties.

Supplements and Vitamins for Autoimmune Disease

Supplements and vitamins play a crucial role in managing autoimmune diseases. Autoimmune diseases occur when the immune system mistakenly attacks the body's own tissues, leading to chronic inflammation and a wide range of symptoms that can significantly impact a person's quality of life. Many people with autoimmune diseases turn to supplements and vitamins as a way to manage their symptoms and improve their overall health.

The right combination of supplements and vitamins can help support the immune system, reduce inflammation, and improve gut health. This can be especially important for people with autoimmune diseases, who often suffer from nutrient deficiencies due to their condition or the medications they take.

Here, we will discuss some of the most effective supplements and vitamins for autoimmune diseases and how they can help manage symptoms and improve overall health.

Vitamin D

Vitamin D is essential for a strong immune system and has been shown to play a role in reducing the risk of autoimmune diseases. This vitamin is commonly referred to as the "sunshine vitamin" because the body can produce it when the skin is exposed to sunlight. However, many people with autoimmune diseases are deficient in vitamin D, which can contribute to their condition.

Studies have shown that supplementing with vitamin D can reduce the severity of autoimmune symptoms and improve overall health. Vitamin D is also important for bone health and can help prevent osteoporosis, a common complication of autoimmune diseases.

Omega-3 Fatty Acids

Omega-3 fatty acids are essential for reducing inflammation and improving overall health. They are found in fatty fish such as salmon, mackerel, and sardines, as well as in supplements like fish oil and krill oil.

Studies have shown that omega-3 fatty acids can improve symptoms in people with autoimmune diseases, including reducing joint pain and swelling, improving skin health, and reducing inflammation in the gut. Omega-3 fatty acids are also important for heart health and can help lower cholesterol levels, which is important for people with autoimmune diseases who are at increased risk for heart disease.

Vitamin B12

Vitamin B12 is essential for proper brain function and the production of red blood cells. People with autoimmune diseases are at increased risk for vitamin B12 deficiency, which can lead to anemia, fatigue, and nerve damage.

Supplementing with vitamin B12 can help improve energy levels and reduce fatigue in people with autoimmune diseases. Vitamin B12 is also important for maintaining healthy nerve function, which can help prevent nerve damage in people with autoimmune diseases.

Probiotics

Probiotics are beneficial bacteria that live in the gut and help support digestive health. People with autoimmune diseases are at increased risk for gut problems, including leaky gut syndrome and gut dysbiosis, which can contribute to their condition.

Supplementing with probiotics can help improve gut health, reduce inflammation, and support the immune system. Probiotics are also important for maintaining a healthy balance of bacteria in the gut, which can help prevent the overgrowth of harmful bacteria that can contribute to autoimmune diseases.

Magnesium

Magnesium is a mineral that is important for many bodily processes, including the production of energy, the functioning of the nervous system, and the regulation of blood sugar levels. People with autoimmune diseases are at increased risk for magnesium deficiency, which can contribute to symptoms such as fatigue, muscle weakness, and insomnia.

Supplementing with magnesium can help improve energy levels, reduce muscle weakness, and improve sleep in people with autoimmune diseases. Magnesium is also important for maintaining healthy bone density, which is important for people with autoimmune diseases who are at increased risk for osteoporosis.

Vitamin C

Vitamin C is a powerful antioxidant that helps support the immune system and reduce inflammation. People with autoimmune diseases are often deficient in vitamin C, which can contribute to their symptoms.

Studies have shown that supplementing with vitamin C can reduce inflammation, improve gut health, and support the immune system in people with autoimmune diseases. Vitamin C is also important for skin health and can help prevent skin damage and improve skin healing in people with autoimmune diseases.

Zinc

Zinc is an essential mineral that is important for immune function and wound healing. People with autoimmune diseases are at increased risk for zinc deficiency, which can contribute to their symptoms.

Supplementing with zinc can help improve immune function, reduce inflammation, and support wound healing in people with autoimmune diseases. Zinc is also important for healthy skin, hair, and nails and can help improve skin health and prevent skin damage in people with autoimmune diseases.

Curcumin

Curcumin is a compound found in turmeric that has powerful anti-inflammatory and antioxidant properties. It has been shown to be effective in managing a wide range of autoimmune diseases, including rheumatoid arthritis, lupus, and Crohn's disease.

Studies have shown that supplementing with curcumin can reduce inflammation, improve gut health, and support the immune system in people with autoimmune diseases. Curcumin is also important for reducing pain and improving joint health in people with autoimmune diseases.

Glutathione

Glutathione is an antioxidant that is important for reducing inflammation and supporting the immune system. People with autoimmune diseases are often deficient in glutathione, which can contribute to their symptoms.

Supplementing with glutathione can help reduce inflammation, improve gut health, and support the immune system in people with autoimmune diseases. Glutathione is also important for reducing oxidative stress and improving overall health in people with autoimmune diseases.

It is important to note that supplements and vitamins should not be used as a substitute for conventional medical treatment for autoimmune diseases. They should only be used in conjunction with a healthy diet and lifestyle changes and under the supervision of a healthcare provider. Additionally, some supplements and vitamins can interact with medications, so it is important to talk to your doctor before starting any new supplement regimen.

The Importance of Probiotics and Fermented Foods

The gut is a vital part of the human body and plays a crucial role in overall health. The gut is home to trillions of microorganisms, including bacteria, yeast, and viruses, collectively known as the gut microbiome.

The gut microbiome is responsible for various functions such as digestion, nutrient absorption, and immune system regulation. It is therefore important to maintain a healthy balance of microorganisms in the gut to ensure optimal health. Probiotics and fermented foods are crucial components in maintaining this balance and have been shown to have numerous health benefits.

What are Probiotics?

Probiotics are live microorganisms that have been shown to have a beneficial effect on the host's health. They are commonly referred to as "good bacteria" and are found in various food and supplement products. Probiotics work by increasing the number of beneficial bacteria in the gut and thereby improving gut health.

They also help to balance the gut microbiome by suppressing the growth of harmful bacteria, thereby improving overall gut health.

Types of Probiotics

The most common types of probiotics are Lactobacillus and Bifid bacterium, which are commonly found in fermented foods such as yogurt and kefir. Other common types of probiotics include Streptococcus thermophiles and Lacto coccus lactic, which are found in dairy products, and Escherichia coli and Bacillus subtilis, which are found in fermented vegetables.

Health Benefits of Probiotics

There are numerous health benefits associated with the consumption of probiotics. Some of the most well-known benefits include:

Improving digestion: Probiotics can improve digestion by increasing the production of digestive enzymes and improving the absorption of nutrients.

They also help to regulate bowel movements, reducing symptoms of constipation and diarrhea.

Boosting the immune system: Probiotics play an important role in boosting the immune system by regulating the gut microbiome and suppressing the growth of harmful bacteria.

Reducing inflammation: Probiotics have anti-inflammatory properties that can help to reduce inflammation throughout the body. This is particularly important in conditions such as irritable bowel syndrome (IBS) and Crohn's disease.

Promoting weight loss: Probiotics have been shown to improve weight loss by reducing the absorption of fat and increasing feelings of fullness.

Improving mental health: Probiotics have been shown to improve mental health by reducing symptoms of depression and anxiety.

Reducing the risk of chronic diseases: Probiotics have been shown to reduce the risk of chronic diseases such as heart disease and type 2 diabetes.

What are Fermented Foods?

Fermented foods are foods that have undergone a process of lacto-fermentation, where bacteria such as Lactobacillus ferment the sugars and carbohydrates in the food.

This process produces lactic acid, which acts as a preservative and helps to increase the shelf-life of the food. Fermented foods are a rich source of probiotics and have been shown to have numerous health benefits.

Types of Fermented Foods

Some of the most common fermented foods include yogurt, kefir, sauerkraut, kimchi, pickles, and miso. Each of these fermented foods is unique in its flavor and nutritional profile, making it easy to incorporate them into a varied diet.

Health Benefits of Fermented Foods

The health benefits of fermented foods are similar to those of probiotics and include:

Improving digestion: Fermented foods help to improve digestion by increasing the production of digestive enzymes and improving the absorption of nutrients. They also help to regulate bowel movements, reducing symptoms of constipation and diarrhea.

Boosting the immune system: Fermented foods play an important role in boosting the immune system by regulating the gut microbiome and suppressing the growth of harmful bacteria.

Reducing inflammation: Fermented foods contain natural anti-inflammatory compounds that can help to reduce inflammation throughout the body. This is particularly important in conditions such as irritable bowel syndrome (IBS) and Crohn's disease.

Promoting weight loss: Fermented foods are low in calories and high in fiber, making them an excellent option for those looking to lose weight.

Improving mental health: Fermented foods have been shown to improve mental health by reducing symptoms of depression and anxiety.

Reducing the risk of chronic diseases: Fermented foods have been shown to reduce the risk of chronic diseases such as heart disease and type 2 diabetes.

How to Incorporate Probiotics and Fermented Foods into Your Diet

Incorporating probiotics and fermented foods into your diet is easy and can be done in several ways. Here are a few simple steps to help you get started:

Eat a variety of fermented foods: Try to include a variety of fermented foods in your diet to ensure that you are getting a wide range of probiotics.

Make your own fermented foods: You can easily make your own fermented foods at home, such as sauerkraut, kimchi, and pickles. This is a great way to save money and ensure that you are getting high-quality, fresh fermented foods.

Choose probiotic-rich foods: Look for foods that are high in probiotics, such as yogurt, kefir, and fermented vegetables.

Take a probiotic supplement: If you are unable to get enough probiotics from your diet, consider taking a probiotic supplement.

The Impact of Healthy Fats on Autoimmune Diseases

Autoimmune diseases, such as rheumatoid arthritis, lupus, and multiple sclerosis, are a group of disorders that occur when the immune system mistakenly attacks healthy tissues in the body. The exact cause of autoimmune diseases is not yet known, but researchers have found that a combination of genetic and environmental factors, such as diet, stress, and toxins, may play a role.

While there is no cure for autoimmune diseases, managing the symptoms and reducing the severity of attacks is crucial for those affected by these conditions. In this article, we will explore the impact of healthy fats on autoimmune diseases and how they can be used as part of a comprehensive treatment plan.

The Importance of Healthy Fats in the Diet

Fat is an essential nutrient that plays a vital role in overall health. It helps to insulate the body, provide energy, and protect the organs. Fat also plays a crucial role in hormone regulation, cell membrane structure, and immune function.

While all fats are important, the type of fat you eat is equally crucial. Saturated and trans fats, often found in processed and junk foods, can increase inflammation in the body and contribute to a wide range of health problems. On the other hand, unsaturated fats, such as omega-3 and omega-6 fatty acids, can have anti-inflammatory effects and provide numerous health benefits.

Healthy Fats and Inflammation

Inflammation is a normal response of the immune system to injury or infection. However, chronic inflammation, which occurs when the immune system is activated for an extended period, can lead to a wide range of health problems, including autoimmune diseases. Chronic inflammation can cause the immune system to attack healthy tissues, leading to the development of autoimmune diseases.

Healthy fats, such as omega-3 and omega-6 fatty acids, have anti-inflammatory effects and can help reduce chronic inflammation in the body. Omega-3 fatty acids, found in fatty fish such as salmon, sardines, and anchovies, as well as flaxseeds, chia seeds, and walnuts, have been shown to reduce inflammation in the body. Omega-3 fatty acids are converted into anti-inflammatory compounds, such as eicosapentaenoic acid (EPA) and docosahexaenoic acid (DHA), which can help reduce inflammation and protect against autoimmune diseases.

Omega-6 fatty acids, found in foods such as sunflower seeds, pumpkin seeds, and almonds, also have anti-inflammatory effects. However, unlike omega-3 fatty acids, they are easily converted into pro-inflammatory compounds if they are consumed in excess. A balanced ratio of omega-3 to omega-6 fatty acids is crucial for reducing inflammation in the body and preventing autoimmune diseases.

Healthy Fats and Immune Function

Fat is a crucial component of cell membranes and plays a role in immune function. The type of fat you eat can have a significant impact on the immune system, with healthy fats helping to improve immune function and reduce the risk of autoimmune diseases.

Omega-3 fatty acids have been shown to improve immune function and reduce the risk of autoimmune diseases. For example, studies have shown that omega-3 fatty acids can improve the function of immune cells, such as T cells and B cells, and reduce the risk of autoimmune diseases.

Omega-6 fatty acids also play a role in immune function, but they are easily converted into pro-inflammatory compounds if they are consumed in excess. A balanced ratio of omega-3 to omega-6 fatty acids is crucial for reducing inflammation and maintaining a healthy immune system.

Healthy Fats and the Gut Microbiome The gut microbiome, the community of microorganisms that live in the gut, plays a crucial role in overall health, including immune function and the development of autoimmune diseases. The type of fat you eat can have a significant impact on the gut microbiome and, in turn, on the risk of autoimmune diseases.

Healthy fats, such as omega-3 fatty acids, have been shown to improve the gut microbiome and reduce the risk of autoimmune diseases. Omega-3 fatty acids have been shown to increase the population of beneficial bacteria in the gut, such as Lactobacillus and Bifid bacterium, and reduce the population of harmful bacteria, such as Escherichia coli. This balance of beneficial and harmful bacteria in the gut is crucial for reducing inflammation and maintaining a healthy immune system.

On the other hand, unhealthy fats, such as Trans and saturated fats, have been shown to negatively impact the gut microbiome and increase the risk of autoimmune diseases. Trans and saturated fats have been shown to increase the population of harmful bacteria in the gut and reduce the population of beneficial bacteria. This imbalance of bacteria in the gut can contribute to chronic inflammation and increase the risk of autoimmune diseases.

Chapter 5: Step 3: Reinoculate

The Importance of Repopulating the Gut with Beneficial Bacteria

The gut is home to trillions of bacteria, some of which are beneficial and some of which are harmful. This complex and delicate ecosystem is known as the gut microbiome and it plays a crucial role in our health and wellbeing.

The gut microbiome influences everything from our digestive function and nutrient absorption to our immune system and mental health. When the gut microbiome is out of balance, it can lead to a range of health problems, including autoimmune diseases, digestive disorders, and mental health issues.

The importance of repopulating the gut with beneficial bacteria lies in the role that these bacteria play in maintaining a healthy gut microbiome. Beneficial bacteria are essential for regulating the balance of bacteria in the gut and keeping harmful bacteria in check. They also help to break down food and absorb nutrients, protect against infections, and produce beneficial compounds that improve our overall health.

Unfortunately, many factors can disrupt the gut microbiome and disrupt the balance of beneficial bacteria. Antibiotics, stress, a poor diet, and environmental toxins are just a few of the factors that can cause an overgrowth of harmful bacteria and lead to an imbalanced gut microbiome. This is why repopulating the gut with beneficial bacteria is so important.

One of the best ways to repopulate the gut with beneficial bacteria is through the use of probiotics. Probiotics are live bacteria and yeasts that are similar to the beneficial bacteria found in the gut. They are available in supplement form or in fermented foods such as yogurt, kefir, sauerkraut, and kombucha. Probiotics help to restore the balance of bacteria in the gut and improve overall gut health.

Another way to repopulate the gut with beneficial bacteria is through the use of prebiotics. Prebiotics are non-digestible fibers that act as food for the beneficial bacteria in the gut. By consuming prebiotics, you are helping to feed the beneficial bacteria and encourage their growth. Foods such as chicory root, garlic, onions, leeks, and asparagus are all rich in prebiotics.

The combination of probiotics and prebiotics is known as a symbiotic. Symbiotic are believed to be even more effective at restoring the balance of bacteria in the gut than probiotics or prebiotics alone. By consuming both probiotics and prebiotics, you are helping to create the ideal environment for beneficial bacteria to thrive.

Another way to repopulate the gut with beneficial bacteria is through the use of fermented foods. Fermented foods are rich in probiotics and have been used for thousands of years to improve gut health. Foods such as yogurt, kefir, sauerkraut, and kombucha are all examples of fermented foods. By incorporating these foods into your diet, you are helping to restore the balance of bacteria in the gut and improve overall gut health.

In addition to repopulating the gut with beneficial bacteria, it is also important to take steps to reduce the number of harmful bacteria in the gut. This includes avoiding antibiotics unless they are absolutely necessary, reducing stress, and eating a diet that is rich in whole, unprocessed foods and low in sugar and refined carbohydrates. By taking these steps, you can help to create a healthy gut environment that is conducive to the growth of beneficial bacteria.

The Role of Probiotics and Fermented Foods

The role of probiotics and fermented foods has become increasingly important in recent years, as more and more people are seeking natural and holistic ways to maintain their health and prevent disease. Probiotics and fermented foods have been shown to have a significant impact on digestive health, as well as a range of other health conditions, including autoimmune diseases, skin disorders, and mental health. In this article, we will explore the role of probiotics and fermented foods in maintaining good health and preventing disease, and the benefits that these foods offer for the gut and overall health.

Probiotics are live microorganisms that are beneficial to the human body. They are commonly found in fermented foods, such as yogurt, kefir, and sauerkraut, and can also be found in supplement form. The human body is home to trillions of bacteria, both good and bad, and the balance between these bacteria is critical for maintaining good health. Probiotics help to promote the growth of good bacteria in the gut, which can help to maintain a healthy gut microbiome and prevent the growth of harmful bacteria.

Fermented foods are foods that have been transformed through the action of microorganisms, such as yeast or bacteria. This process of fermentation helps to preserve the food and increases its nutritional value by producing beneficial bacteria, enzymes, and vitamins. The most well-known fermented food is yogurt, but there are many other fermented foods that offer similar benefits, including kefir, sauerkraut, kimchi, miso, and kombucha.

The gut microbiome plays a critical role in maintaining good health and preventing disease. The gut microbiome is made up of trillions of bacteria, fungi, and viruses that live in the digestive tract and help to regulate the body's functions. The balance between the good and bad bacteria in the gut microbiome is critical for maintaining good health, and an imbalance of bacteria can lead to a range of health conditions, including autoimmune diseases, skin disorders, and mental health issues.

Probiotics and fermented foods have been shown to have a significant impact on the gut microbiome, and can help to promote the growth of good bacteria and prevent the growth of harmful bacteria. This can help to maintain a healthy gut microbiome and prevent a range of health conditions.

For example, research has shown that probiotics and fermented foods can help to improve digestive health by reducing symptoms of irritable bowel syndrome (IBS), reducing bloating, and improving gut motility.

In addition to digestive health, probiotics and fermented foods have also been shown to have a positive impact on the skin. The skin is an important barrier that helps to protect the body from harmful substances, and the gut microbiome plays a critical role in maintaining healthy skin. Probiotics and fermented foods can help to maintain the balance of bacteria in the gut microbiome, which can help to prevent skin conditions such as acne, eczema, and psoriasis.

Mental health is another area where probiotics and fermented foods have been shown to have a positive impact. The gut microbiome has been shown to play a critical role in mental health, and an imbalance of bacteria in the gut microbiome has been linked to a range of mental health conditions, including anxiety and depression.

Probiotics and fermented foods can help to promote the growth of good bacteria in the gut, which can help to improve mental health and reduce the risk of mental health conditions.

The Benefits of Prebiotics And Symbiotic

Prebiotics and symbiotic are two related but distinct components of gut health that have been shown to offer a wide range of health benefits. Prebiotics are non-digestible fibers that feed the beneficial bacteria in our gut, while symbiotic are a combination of prebiotics and probiotics. In this article, we will explore the benefits of prebiotics and symbiotic and why they are essential for maintaining a healthy gut.

First, let's examine the role of prebiotics in our gut. Prebiotics are types of fiber that are not digested by our digestive enzymes. Instead, they pass through our gut and provide a source of food for the beneficial bacteria that live there. This beneficial bacteria are known as probiotics, and they play a critical role in maintaining gut health. By providing these probiotics with a source of nutrition, prebiotics help to promote the growth and reproduction of these beneficial bacteria. This, in turn, helps to maintain a healthy gut microbiome, which is critical for overall health and well-being.

One of the most significant benefits of prebiotics is their ability to improve gut health. A healthy gut microbiome is critical for maintaining a healthy digestive system. The beneficial bacteria in our gut play a key role in breaking down and digesting our food, as well as absorbing nutrients and producing important compounds like vitamins and short-chain fatty acids.

By feeding these bacteria with prebiotics, we help to promote a healthy gut microbiome, which can help to prevent digestive issues like bloating, constipation, and diarrhea.

Another important benefit of prebiotics is their ability to boost the immune system. Our gut microbiome is critical for our overall health, and it plays a key role in regulating our immune system. When our gut microbiome is healthy and balanced, it helps to prevent infections and diseases. By feeding the beneficial bacteria in our gut with prebiotics, we can help to improve our immune system and reduce the risk of infection and disease.

Prebiotics are also known for their ability to reduce inflammation in the gut. Chronic inflammation is a key contributor to many autoimmune diseases, as well as a wide range of other health issues, including heart disease and cancer. By feeding the beneficial bacteria in our gut with prebiotics, we can help to reduce inflammation in the gut and reduce the risk of these diseases.

Prebiotics are also beneficial for our mental health. Recent research has shown that the gut microbiome plays a critical role in our mental health and well-being. The beneficial bacteria in our gut produce important compounds like serotonin, which helps to regulate our mood, and improve our mental health. By feeding these bacteria with prebiotics, we can help to improve our mental health and reduce the risk of mental health issues like depression and anxiety.

Now, let's turn our attention to symbiotic. Symbiotic are a combination of prebiotics and probiotics, and they offer a range of benefits that go beyond what prebiotics and probiotics can provide on their own. By combining these two components, symbiotic help to create a symbiotic relationship between the beneficial bacteria in our gut and the prebiotics that feed them. This, in turn, helps to promote the growth and reproduction of the beneficial bacteria, and to maintain a healthy gut microbiome.

One of the key benefits of symbiotic is their ability to improve gut health. As we have already discussed, a healthy gut microbiome is critical for maintaining a healthy digestive system. By combining prebiotics and probiotics in a symbiotic formula, we can help to promote the growth and reproduction of the beneficial bacteria in our gut, and to maintain a healthy gut microbiome. This, in turn, can help to prevent digestive issues, improve nutrient absorption, and support overall gut health.

Another benefit of symbiotic is their ability to enhance the immune system. The gut microbiome is critical for regulating the immune system, and by feeding the beneficial bacteria with prebiotics and providing them with probiotics, we can help to improve the immune system and reduce the risk of infections and diseases. This is particularly important for individuals who are susceptible to infections or have a weakened immune system, as symbiotic can help to support and enhance their immune system function.

Symbiotic can also help to reduce inflammation in the gut. Chronic inflammation is a major contributor to many health issues, including autoimmune diseases and digestive problems. By combining prebiotics and probiotics, symbiotic can help to reduce inflammation in the gut and improve gut health. This can help to reduce the risk of these health problems and promote overall well-being.

In addition to their health benefits, symbiotic are also beneficial for weight management. Recent research has shown that the gut microbiome plays a critical role in weight regulation and metabolism. By maintaining a healthy gut microbiome with symbiotic, we can help to regulate our weight, reduce the risk of obesity, and improve overall health and wellness.

Chapter 6: Step 4: Repair

The Importance of Repairing the Gut Lining

The gut lining is an incredibly important part of the human body and is responsible for many essential functions. It acts as a barrier between the inside of the gut and the rest of the body, protecting against harmful substances and ensuring that essential nutrients are absorbed into the bloodstream.

However, when the gut lining becomes damaged, it can lead to a range of serious health problems, including autoimmune diseases, food sensitivities, and chronic inflammation. This is why repairing the gut lining is so important, and should be a key part of any holistic approach to health and wellness.

The gut lining is made up of a single layer of cells that are closely packed together, with tiny spaces between them. This barrier is designed to allow essential nutrients and fluids to pass through, while preventing harmful substances from entering the bloodstream. The gut lining is held together by tight junctions, which are made up of proteins that form a barrier between the cells. When these tight junctions become damaged, they can no longer provide an effective barrier, which can lead to a range of health problems.

One of the main causes of gut lining damage is inflammation. Inflammation is a natural response of the body to injury or infection, but when it becomes chronic, it can cause significant damage to the gut lining. Chronic inflammation can be caused by a variety of factors, including a poor diet, stress, and exposure to toxins. When the gut lining becomes inflamed, it can cause the tight junctions to loosen, which can lead to a leaky gut.

A leaky gut is a condition where the gut lining becomes permeable, allowing harmful substances to enter the bloodstream. This can lead to a range of symptoms, including bloating, abdominal pain, and fatigue. In addition, a leaky gut can also increase the risk of developing autoimmune diseases, as the immune system becomes more likely to attack the body's own tissues.

The good news is that the gut lining can be repaired, and there are many natural and effective ways to do this. One of the most important things that you can do is to adopt a healthy, balanced diet that is rich in nutrient-dense foods. This includes plenty of fresh fruits and vegetables, whole grains, lean protein, and healthy fats. In addition, it is important to limit your intake of processed foods and sugar, as these can contribute to inflammation and damage the gut lining.

How to heal the gut lining through diet and supplements

The gut lining is a delicate and complex system that is responsible for maintaining good health. When the gut lining is damaged, it can lead to a number of health problems, including autoimmune diseases, allergies, and digestive disorders. In order to heal the gut lining and prevent further damage, it is important to make changes to your diet and consider taking specific supplements.

One of the most important steps in healing the gut lining is to remove foods and substances that can cause damage. This includes foods that are high in lectins, such as grains and legumes, and foods that contain gluten. Gluten is a protein found in wheat, barley, and rye, and is known to cause damage to the gut lining. Additionally, it is important to eliminate sugar and processed foods, as these can feed harmful bacteria in the gut and cause further damage.

In addition to removing damaging foods and substances, it is important to replace them with nutrient-dense foods that are rich in vitamins and minerals. This includes eating plenty of leafy greens, healthy fats, and lean protein. Leafy greens are rich in antioxidants and fiber, which can help to heal the gut lining and prevent further damage. Healthy fats, such as omega-3 fatty acids, can help to reduce inflammation and improve gut health. Lean protein, such as chicken and fish, can help to support the growth of beneficial bacteria in the gut.

Another important step in healing the gut lining is to reinoculate the gut with beneficial bacteria. This can be achieved by taking probiotics and eating fermented foods, such as kefir, kimchi, and sauerkraut. Probiotics are beneficial bacteria that can help to support the growth of healthy gut bacteria, while fermented foods are a natural source of probiotics. By reinoculating the gut with beneficial bacteria, you can help to improve gut health and support the healing process.

Finally, it is important to repair the gut lining through the use of specific supplements. One of the most important supplements for gut health is L-glutamine, an amino acid that can help to support the growth of healthy gut cells and reduce inflammation. Additionally, it is important to take a high-quality, multi-strain probiotic supplement to support the growth of beneficial bacteria in the gut. Other supplements that can be helpful for gut health include omega-3 fatty acids, vitamin D, and aloe vera.

The Role of Probiotics, Prebiotics, and Symbiotic

The role of probiotics, prebiotics, and symbiotic has become increasingly important in recent years as researchers have uncovered the crucial role that gut health plays in overall health and wellness. These three terms are often used interchangeably, but they actually refer to distinct components of gut health that work together to support the health of the gut microbiome.

Understanding the difference between these terms is critical to understanding how they can be used to promote good gut health.

Probiotics are live microorganisms that can be consumed in food or supplements to promote the health of the gut microbiome. These microorganisms are typically bacteria, but they can also be yeast or other organisms. Probiotics are beneficial because they help to maintain the balance of microorganisms in the gut, which is essential for overall health and wellness. When the balance of microorganisms in the gut is disrupted, it can lead to a variety of health problems, including digestive issues, inflammation, and autoimmune diseases.

Prebiotics are non-digestible food ingredients that are designed to nourish the beneficial bacteria in the gut. These ingredients provide fuel for the probiotics, allowing them to grow and multiply, which can help to maintain the balance of microorganisms in the gut. Prebiotics can be found in a variety of foods, including fiber-rich foods such as fruits, vegetables, and whole grains. Some common prebiotics include inulin, fructooligosaccharides (FOS), and galactooligosaccharides (GOS).

Symbiotic are a combination of probiotics and prebiotics, designed to work together to promote gut health. Symbiotic are thought to be more effective than either probiotics or prebiotics alone because they help to maintain the balance of microorganisms in the gut, while also providing the probiotics with the nutrients they need to thrive. There are a variety of symbiotic products available, including supplements and fermented foods, such as yogurt and kefir.

The role of probiotics in gut health is well-established, and they have been used for centuries as a way to promote gut health and treat digestive issues. For example, fermented foods like yogurt and kefir have been used for centuries as a way to promote gut health, and modern research has confirmed that these foods contain probiotics that are beneficial for the gut.

In addition to promoting gut health, probiotics have been shown to have a variety of other health benefits, including:

- Reducing inflammation
- Improving immune function
- Reducing the symptoms of certain autoimmune diseases
- Supporting mental health and reducing symptoms of anxiety and depression
- Supporting weight management
- Improving skin health

Prebiotics are also essential for good gut health, as they provide fuel for the probiotics, allowing them to grow and multiply. Prebiotics have also been shown to have a variety of health benefits, including:

- Improving gut health by promoting the growth of beneficial bacteria
- Reducing inflammation
- Improving insulin sensitivity and reducing the risk of type 2 diabetes
- Improving immune function
- Supporting weight management
- Improving heart health

The combination of probiotics and prebiotics in symbiotic has been shown to be even more effective than either probiotics or prebiotics alone. This is because symbiotic provide the probiotics with the nutrients they need to thrive, while also helping to maintain the balance of microorganisms in the gut.

One of the most important benefits of symbiotic is their ability to improve gut health by promoting the growth of beneficial bacteria. This is essential for maintaining the balance of microorganisms in the gut, which is crucial for overall health and wellness. When the balance of micro organisms in the gut is disrupted, it can lead to a variety of health problems, including digestive issues, inflammation, and autoimmune diseases. By promoting the growth of beneficial bacteria, symbiotic can help to improve gut health and reduce the risk of these health problems.

In addition to improving gut health, symbiotic have also been shown to have a variety of other health benefits, including:

- Reducing inflammation
- Improving immune function
- Reducing symptoms of certain autoimmune diseases

- Improving mental health and reducing symptoms of anxiety and depression

- Supporting weight management

- Improving skin health

It is important to note that not all probiotics, prebiotics, and symbiotic are created equal. The specific strain of probiotic, the type of prebiotic, and the combination of probiotics and prebiotics in symbiotic can all play a role in the health benefits they provide. Therefore, it is important to choose high-quality products that have been well-researched and have been shown to provide health benefits.

The Impact of Lifestyle Changes on Gut Healing

The gut microbiome is a complex network of microorganisms that play a crucial role in maintaining gut health. These microorganisms help in breaking down food, producing essential vitamins and nutrients, and keeping harmful pathogens at bay. The gut microbiome is easily impacted by lifestyle factors, and a disrupted gut microbiome can lead to numerous health problems such as allergies, autoimmune diseases, and digestive issues.

One of the most significant lifestyle factors that can impact the gut is diet. The gut microbiome is highly sensitive to the foods that an individual consumes, and a diet that is high in processed foods, sugar, and unhealthy fats can have a detrimental impact on the gut. Such a diet can lead to an overgrowth of harmful bacteria and yeast, which can disrupt the delicate balance of the gut microbiome and lead to digestive problems such as bloating, constipation, and diarrhea.

Stress is another lifestyle factor that can impact the gut. Chronic stress can lead to inflammation and damage to the gut lining, which can make it more permeable and susceptible to harmful pathogens. This can also cause an overgrowth of harmful bacteria and yeast, leading to digestive problems and other health issues. To combat the effects of stress, individuals can adopt stress-management techniques such as mindfulness, exercise, and relaxation.

Physical activity is also essential for maintaining gut health. Exercise helps in reducing stress, improving circulation, and increasing the production of beneficial gut bacteria. A sedentary lifestyle, on the other hand, can lead to decreased gut mobility and a sluggish digestive system, which can lead to digestive problems. Regular physical activity, even as simple as a brisk walk, can help in improving gut health.

Exposure to chemicals and toxins can also impact gut health. These toxins can come from various sources, including personal care products, cleaning products, and food preservatives. Toxins can disrupt the gut microbiome, causing an overgrowth of harmful bacteria and yeast, and leading to digestive problems and other health issues. To reduce exposure to toxins, individuals can switch to natural, chemical-free products and avoid processed foods that contain preservatives and other harmful chemicals.

Chapter 7: Implementing the Autoimmune Solution

How to put the autoimmune solution into action

Putting the autoimmune solution into action can be a challenging and overwhelming process for those who are new to the idea. However, with proper guidance and a solid plan in place, it is possible to effectively prevent and reverse autoimmune diseases. In this article, we will explore the steps that individuals can take to put the autoimmune solution into action and achieve optimal health.

The first step in putting the autoimmune solution into action is to identify and remove autoimmune triggers. This includes common allergens such as gluten, dairy, soy, and corn, as well as environmental irritants like chemicals and pollutants. It is important to eliminate these triggers from the diet and environment to prevent the immune system from attacking the body. A comprehensive food elimination program can be a great place to start. This may include following a strict autoimmune protocol diet, which removes all potentially problematic foods, or working with a functional medicine practitioner to determine which triggers may be specific to an individual.

The second step in putting the autoimmune solution into action is to replace harmful foods and chemicals with nutrient-dense, whole foods. This includes eating a variety of fresh fruits and vegetables, lean proteins, and healthy fats, such as those found in avocados, nuts, and seeds. It is also important to incorporate fermented foods, such as kimchi, sauerkraut, and kefir, into the diet to support gut health. In addition, a high-quality multivitamin,

vitamin D, and Omega-3 supplements can help support the immune system and provide additional nutrients that may be lacking in the diet.

The third step in putting the autoimmune solution into action is to reinoculate the gut with beneficial bacteria. This is achieved through the consumption of probiotics, prebiotics, and symbiotic. Probiotics are live bacteria that can be found in fermented foods or taken as supplements. Prebiotics are indigestible fibers that feed the beneficial bacteria in the gut, while symbiotic are a combination of probiotics and prebiotics. These three components work together to support the gut microbiome and promote a healthy balance of bacteria in the gut.

The final step in putting the autoimmune solution into action is to repair the gut lining. This involves addressing the underlying cause of gut inflammation and promoting gut healing. This can be achieved through diet, lifestyle changes, and supplements. For example, incorporating bone broth into the diet can help to heal the gut lining, as can avoiding processed foods, eating a variety of nutrient-dense foods, and managing stress levels. Additionally, supplements like L-glutamine, N-acetyl glucosamine, and zinc can support gut healing and help to reduce inflammation.

It is important to monitor progress throughout the autoimmune solution program and make any necessary adjustments. This may involve working with a functional medicine practitioner or nutritionist who can help track progress and provide support. Keeping a journal of symptoms and diet can also be a helpful tool in tracking progress and identifying potential triggers.

In addition to dietary and lifestyle changes, it is important to incorporate stress management techniques into the autoimmune solution program. This may include practicing mindfulness, meditation, or yoga, as well as engaging in regular physical activity. Managing stress levels can help to prevent flare-ups and improve overall health.

The Role of Lifestyle Changes

Lifestyle changes are a critical component of preventing and reversing autoimmune diseases. The importance of incorporating healthy habits into daily life cannot be overstated, as they have a significant impact on the functioning of the immune system and overall health. In this article, we will explore the role of lifestyle changes in autoimmune diseases and the benefits of making these changes.

Autoimmune diseases are conditions in which the body's immune system mistakenly attacks its own tissues, leading to inflammation and tissue damage. The exact causes of autoimmune diseases are still not fully understood, but genetics, environmental factors, gut health, and stress are all known to play a role.

Lifestyle changes, such as diet and exercise, have been shown to have a significant impact on autoimmune diseases. For example, research has shown that following a healthy diet rich in nutrient-dense foods and avoiding processed foods and chemicals can help to reduce inflammation in the body and improve gut health. Similarly, regular exercise has been shown to help reduce stress and improve overall health, which can in turn help to prevent and reverse autoimmune diseases.

One of the key ways that lifestyle changes can impact autoimmune diseases is through the gut-immune connection. The gut is home to trillions of bacteria, known as the gut microbiome, which play a critical role in the functioning of the immune system. Research has shown that an imbalanced gut microbiome can lead to inflammation in the body, which is a key factor in the development of autoimmune diseases.

By making lifestyle changes, such as incorporating probiotics and fermented foods into the diet and avoiding processed foods and chemicals, individuals can help to improve gut health and balance the gut microbiome. This, in turn, can help to reduce inflammation and prevent the development of autoimmune diseases.

In addition to diet and exercise, stress management is also an important aspect of lifestyle changes for individuals with autoimmune diseases. Stress has been shown to have a negative impact on the immune system, leading to increased inflammation and a heightened risk of autoimmune diseases.

Incorporating stress-management techniques, such as mindfulness, deep breathing, and yoga, can help to reduce stress levels and improve overall health. Additionally, getting adequate sleep and engaging in regular physical activity can also help to reduce stress and improve overall health.

Overall, lifestyle changes play a critical role in preventing and reversing autoimmune diseases. By incorporating healthy habits into daily life, individuals can help to improve their gut health, reduce inflammation, and reduce stress levels, all of which can have a positive impact on autoimmune diseases.

It is important to note that lifestyle changes are not a cure for autoimmune diseases, but they can help to manage symptoms and improve overall health. Individuals with autoimmune diseases should always work with their healthcare provider to develop an individualized plan for managing their condition.

The Importance of Monitoring Progress and Making Adjustments

Monitoring progress and making adjustments are crucial steps in any health and wellness journey. In the case of autoimmune diseases, the process of preventing and reversing these conditions requires a concerted effort and a dedicated commitment to change. The autoimmune solution is a four-step program that aims to remove autoimmune triggers, replace them with nutrient-dense foods, reinoculate the gut with beneficial bacteria, and repair the gut lining. Implementing this program is an ongoing process that requires monitoring progress and making adjustments along the way.

The autoimmune solution is designed to be flexible and adaptable to individual needs and circumstances. Monitoring progress allows individuals to see how their bodies are responding to the changes they are making and make any necessary adjustments. This process helps ensure that the program is working effectively and that individuals are on the right track towards preventing and reversing autoimmune diseases.

One of the key components of monitoring progress is tracking symptoms. Individuals who are implementing the autoimmune solution should track any changes in their symptoms, including any improvements or new symptoms that arise. Tracking symptoms can help individuals identify any autoimmune triggers that may be causing a flare-up or worsening of symptoms. This information can then be used to make adjustments to the program, such as avoiding certain foods or increasing the frequency of probiotics.

Another important aspect of monitoring progress is tracking dietary changes. Individuals who are implementing the autoimmune solution should keep a food diary and track what they are eating, how much they are eating, and how they feel after eating. Tracking dietary changes helps individuals identify any foods that may be causing symptoms and make any necessary adjustments to their diet.

Physical activity and exercise are also important aspects of monitoring progress. Individuals who are implementing the autoimmune solution should track their physical activity levels and monitor any changes in their energy levels or symptoms. If individuals experience any symptoms or flares after exercising, they should make adjustments to their exercise regimen.

Monitoring progress also involves tracking any changes in mood or emotional well-being. Individuals who are implementing the autoimmune solution should monitor their stress levels and any changes in their emotional well-being. Stress is a known trigger for autoimmune diseases, and managing stress is an important part of the autoimmune solution. If individuals experience any changes in their emotional well-being, they should make adjustments to their stress management strategies.

Finally, monitoring progress involves tracking progress towards specific goals. Individuals who are implementing the autoimmune solution should set specific goals and track their progress towards achieving these goals. This can include goals related to weight loss, improved energy levels, reduced symptoms, or improved gut health. Tracking progress towards these goals helps individuals stay motivated and on track with the program.

Making adjustments is a crucial part of the autoimmune solution. As individuals monitor their progress, they may need to make adjustments to their program to ensure that they are on the right track towards preventing and reversing autoimmune diseases. These adjustments can include changes to their diet, physical activity levels, stress management strategies, and supplement regimen.

For example, if individuals experience a flare-up of symptoms after eating a certain food, they may need to make adjustments to their diet and avoid that food. If individuals experience a flare-up after a period of high stress, they may need to make adjustments to their stress management strategies. If individuals experience a flare-up after starting a new supplement, they may need to make adjustments to their supplement regimen.

Making adjustments is an ongoing process that requires patience and dedication. Individuals who are implementing the autoimmune solution should not be discouraged if they need to make adjustments to their program. The key is to stay focused on the goal of preventing and reversing autoimmune diseases and to be persistent in the effort to make necessary changes.

Chapter 8: The Autoimmune Solution and Autoimmune Diseases

How the Autoimmune Solution Applies To Different Autoimmune Diseases

The autoimmune solution is a revolutionary approach to preventing and reversing autoimmune diseases. This solution involves four key steps: removing autoimmune triggers, replacing with nutrient-dense foods and supplements, reinoculating with beneficial bacteria, and repairing the gut lining. Each of these steps is designed to address the root causes of autoimmune diseases, including environmental factors, gut health, and lifestyle factors.

However, the autoimmune solution does not just apply to autoimmune diseases in general, but can also be tailored to specific autoimmune diseases. In this chapter, we will explore how the autoimmune solution applies to different autoimmune diseases, including rheumatoid arthritis, lupus, multiple sclerosis, and celiac disease.

Rheumatoid Arthritis

Rheumatoid arthritis is a chronic autoimmune disease that causes inflammation in the joints. The autoimmune solution can help people with rheumatoid arthritis by addressing the root causes of inflammation. Removing autoimmune triggers can help to reduce the body's immune response, reducing inflammation. Replacing with nutrient-dense foods and supplements can also help to reduce inflammation, as well as providing the nutrients the body needs to function optimally. Reinoculating with beneficial bacteria can help to balance the gut microbiome, reducing inflammation and improving overall gut health. Repairing the gut lining is also important for reducing inflammation, as the gut lining acts as a barrier between the body and the outside world.

It is also important to note that people with rheumatoid arthritis should avoid processed foods and chemicals, as they can trigger autoimmune responses and exacerbate symptoms. Additionally, people with rheumatoid arthritis should aim to consume a diet that is rich in anti-inflammatory foods, such as leafy greens, nuts, and fatty fish. Supplements such as turmeric, ginger, and omega-3 fatty acids may also help to reduce inflammation and improve joint health.

Lupus

Lupus is a chronic autoimmune disease that affects multiple organ systems, including the skin, joints, and organs. The autoimmune solution can help people with lupus by addressing the root causes of autoimmune diseases and reducing autoimmune responses. Removing autoimmune triggers can help to reduce the body's immune response, reducing inflammation and the risk of flare-ups.

Replacing with nutrient-dense foods and supplements can also help to reduce inflammation, as well as providing the nutrients the body needs to function optimally. Reinoculating with beneficial bacteria can help to balance the gut microbiome, reducing inflammation and improving overall gut health. Repairing the gut lining is also important for reducing inflammation, as the gut lining acts as a barrier between the body and the outside world.

It is also important to note that people with lupus should avoid processed foods and chemicals, as they can trigger autoimmune responses and exacerbate symptoms. Additionally, people with lupus should aim to consume a diet that is rich in anti-inflammatory foods, such as leafy greens, nuts, and fatty fish. Supplements such as turmeric, ginger, and omega-3 fatty acids may also help to reduce inflammation and improve overall health.

Multiple Sclerosis

Multiple sclerosis is a chronic autoimmune disease that affects the central nervous system. The autoimmune solution can help people with multiple sclerosis by addressing the root causes of autoimmune diseases and reducing autoimmune responses. Removing autoimmune triggers can help to reduce the body's immune response, reducing inflammation and the risk of flare-ups. Replacing with nutrient-dense foods and supplements can also help to reduce inflammation, as well as providing the nutrients the body needs to function optimally. Reinoculating with beneficial bacteria can help to balance the gut microbiome, reducing inflammation and improving overall gut health. Repairing the gut lining is also important for reducing inflammation, as the gut lining acts as a barrier between the body and the outside world.

It is also important for people with multiple sclerosis to avoid processed foods and chemicals, as they can trigger autoimmune responses and exacerbate symptoms. Additionally, people with multiple sclerosis should aim to consume a diet that is rich in anti-inflammatory foods, such as leafy greens, nuts, and fatty fish. Supplements such as turmeric, ginger, and omega-3 fatty acids may also help to reduce inflammation and improve overall health.

In addition, exercise and stress management can also play a significant role in managing symptoms of multiple sclerosis. Regular physical activity, such as yoga, walking, or swimming, can help to improve mobility, reduce fatigue, and manage stress levels.

Celiac Disease

Celiac disease is a chronic autoimmune disease that affects the small intestine. People with celiac disease are intolerant to gluten, a protein found in wheat, barley, and rye. The autoimmune solution can help people with celiac disease by removing autoimmune triggers and promoting a gluten-free diet.

Replacing with nutrient-dense foods and supplements can also help to provide the nutrients the body needs to function optimally, while reinoculating with beneficial bacteria can help to balance the gut microbiome and improve overall gut health. Repairing the gut lining is also important for reducing inflammation, as the gut lining acts as a barrier between the body and the outside world.

It is also important for people with celiac disease to avoid processed foods and chemicals, as they can trigger autoimmune responses and exacerbate symptoms. Additionally, people with celiac disease should aim to consume a diet that is rich in nutrient-dense foods, such as vegetables, fruits, and lean protein sources.

Supplements such as probiotics, Vitamin D, and calcium may also be necessary for those with celiac disease, as the disease can lead to deficiencies in these important nutrients.

Specific Dietary and Lifestyle Recommendations for Autoimmune Diseases

Dietary changes can play a critical role in managing autoimmune diseases. A diet that is rich in anti-inflammatory foods and low in processed and refined foods can help to reduce symptoms and prevent further damage. It is important to avoid common allergens and irritants, such as gluten and dairy, as these can trigger inflammation and worsen symptoms.

One of the most effective diets for managing autoimmune diseases is the autoimmune protocol (AIP) diet. This diet focuses on eliminating inflammatory foods, such as grains, legumes, and processed foods, and replacing them with nutrient-dense foods, such as vegetables, fruits, and healthy fats. The AIP diet also emphasizes the importance of gut healing foods, such as bone broth, fermented foods, and probiotics, as the gut is often at the root of autoimmune diseases.

In addition to dietary changes, lifestyle modifications can also play a critical role in managing autoimmune diseases. Stress management is an essential part of any autoimmune disease management plan. Chronic stress can trigger inflammation and worsen symptoms, so it is important to find ways to manage stress and reduce its impact on the body. This can include activities such as meditation, yoga, and exercise.

Exercise is another important aspect of managing autoimmune diseases. Regular exercise can help to reduce inflammation and improve overall health. However, it is important to choose activities that are low-impact and do not cause unnecessary stress on the body. Gentle activities, such as yoga, walking, and swimming, are recommended for those with autoimmune diseases.

Sleep is also an important part of any autoimmune disease management plan. Getting enough sleep can help to reduce inflammation and improve overall health. Aim for at least 7-9 hours of sleep each night and try to establish a consistent sleep schedule.

In addition to dietary and lifestyle changes, supplements can also play a critical role in managing autoimmune diseases. Vitamin D, omega-3 fatty acids, and probiotics are all supplements that have been shown to have a positive impact on autoimmune diseases. It is important to speak with a healthcare professional before starting any new supplement regimen, as some supplements may interact with medications or have other side effects.

There are specific dietary and lifestyle recommendations for each type of autoimmune disease. For example, those with rheumatoid arthritis may benefit from a diet that is rich in omega-3 fatty acids, while those with lupus may benefit from a diet that is low in processed and refined foods.

Chapter 9: Living with Autoimmune Diseases

The Challenges of Living with Autoimmune Diseases

Living with autoimmune diseases can be an immense challenge, both physically and mentally. These conditions, which occur when the body's immune system mistakenly attacks healthy cells and tissues, can cause a wide range of symptoms, including fatigue, pain, and joint stiffness, to name just a few. However, while the physical symptoms can be difficult to manage, they are only part of the story. There are many other challenges that come with living with autoimmune diseases, and they can be just as difficult to navigate.

One of the first challenges that people with autoimmune diseases face is getting a proper diagnosis. Despite the prevalence of autoimmune diseases, many doctors are not well-versed in their diagnosis and treatment, and some may even dismiss a patient's symptoms as being "all in their head." This can lead to long delays in getting a proper diagnosis, during which time the disease continues to progress and cause more damage to the body.

Once a diagnosis has been made, the next challenge is finding an effective treatment. While there are many medications and treatments available for autoimmune diseases, not all of them are effective for every person, and some can cause serious side effects. This means that finding the right treatment can be a long and difficult process, with many people trying multiple treatments before finding something that works for them.

In addition to the physical challenges, autoimmune diseases can also have a profound impact on a person's mental health. People with autoimmune diseases are at a higher risk of depression and anxiety, as they deal with the constant physical pain and fatigue that comes with these conditions. They may also face discrimination and stigma from others, who may not understand the severity of the disease, or who may judge them for "not being able to handle their own problems." This can lead to feelings of isolation and loneliness, further compounding the mental health struggles that people with autoimmune diseases face.

Another challenge of living with autoimmune diseases is the impact that it can have on daily life. People with autoimmune diseases may not be able to work or participate in activities that they once enjoyed, which can lead to feelings of loss and frustration. They may also face financial difficulties, as medical bills and treatments can be expensive, and insurance may not cover all of the costs. This can add stress and strain to an already challenging situation.

Finally, people with autoimmune diseases may also have to face the difficulty of managing their symptoms on a day-to-day basis. This can involve sticking to strict diets, taking multiple medications, and making lifestyle changes, such as giving up alcohol or reducing stress. For many people, these changes can be difficult to make, especially if they have been a part of their daily routine for a long time.

Living with autoimmune diseases can be a challenging and difficult experience, but it is important to remember that you are not alone. There are many support groups and resources available to help you manage your symptoms and find the right treatment. It is also important to take care of yourself both physically and mentally, and to reach out to friends and family for support. With the right tools and resources, you can learn to manage your autoimmune diseases and lead a fulfilling life.

The Importance of Self-Care and Stress Management

Self-care and stress management are two critical components of a healthy and fulfilling life. In today's fast-paced and highly demanding world, it is essential to prioritize one's well-being and mental health. With the increasing number of stress-related illnesses and the mounting pressures of daily life, taking care of oneself has become more critical than ever before.

Self-care refers to the intentional and deliberate acts one engages in to promote their well-being, both physically and mentally. It includes taking care of one's health, such as eating well, exercising, and getting enough rest, as well as engaging in activities that bring joy, peace, and relaxation, such as meditation, yoga, or spending time with loved ones.

On the other hand, stress management refers to the methods and techniques one uses to reduce the effects of stress and promote well-being. Stress can take a toll on our physical, emotional, and mental health, and if left unchecked, can lead to various health problems, including depression, anxiety, and heart disease.

The importance of self-care and stress management cannot be overstated, especially in our fast-paced, modern lives. Here are a few reasons why prioritizing these practices is essential for overall health and happiness:

Reduces the risk of physical and mental health problems: Prolonged stress can lead to various physical and mental health problems, including depression, anxiety, heart disease, and more. Engaging in self-care and stress management practices can help reduce the effects of stress and prevent these conditions from developing.

Improves mental clarity and focus: When we are stressed, it can be challenging to focus and think clearly. By engaging in self-care and stress management practices, we can reduce stress levels and improve our ability to think and focus, making it easier to tackle daily tasks and responsibilities.

Enhances relationships: When we are stressed and overwhelmed, our relationships can suffer. Engaging in self-care and stress management practices can help us become more patient, understanding, and compassionate, improving our relationships with others.

Promotes happiness and well-being: Self-care and stress management practices can help promote happiness and overall well-being by reducing stress levels, improving mood, and helping us feel more relaxed and centered.

Increases resilience: The world is full of challenges and obstacles, but engaging in self-care and stress management practices can help build resilience and the ability to cope with stress and adversity.

So, how can one prioritize self-care and stress management in their daily lives? Here are a few tips to help:

Prioritize self-care activities: Make time for self-care activities, such as exercise, meditation, or spending time with loved ones. These activities can help reduce stress levels and promote well-being.

Engage in stress-reducing activities: Engage in activities that help reduce stress, such as yoga, deep breathing exercises, or journaling. These practices can help calm the mind and reduce stress levels.

Get enough sleep: Getting enough restful sleep is essential for reducing stress and promoting well-being. Aim to get seven to eight hours of sleep each night.

Practice good nutrition: A healthy, balanced diet can help reduce stress levels and promote physical and mental well-being. Avoid junk food, caffeine, and sugar, and aim to eat plenty of fruits, vegetables, and whole grains.

Stay organized: Being organized can help reduce stress levels and make it easier to manage daily tasks and responsibilities. Create a schedule, make to-do lists, and prioritize tasks to help stay on top of everything.

How to Manage Symptoms and Stay Healthy

One of the most important aspects of managing symptoms and staying healthy is to understand your triggers. Every person with autoimmune diseases is unique, and what triggers symptoms for one person may not affect another. Common triggers include stress, poor nutrition, lack of sleep, exposure to toxins, and infections. By keeping a journal of your symptoms and activities, you can start to identify patterns and determine what triggers your symptoms.

Once you know your triggers, you can take steps to avoid them. This may include reducing stress, eating a balanced and nutrient-dense diet, and avoiding exposure to toxins. It's also important to get adequate sleep, exercise regularly, and engage in activities that promote relaxation and well-being.

In addition to avoiding triggers, it's important to manage symptoms when they do occur. This may include using medications, supplements, and other treatments prescribed by your doctor. However, there are also natural remedies that can help relieve symptoms and promote overall health. For example, many people find relief from symptoms such as pain, fatigue, and anxiety with practices such as meditation, yoga, and acupuncture.

It's also essential to maintain a positive outlook and take care of your mental health. Chronic diseases can take a toll on your mental well-being, but it's important to remember that you're not alone. Joining a support group, seeking therapy, and engaging in activities that bring you joy can help improve your mental health and reduce symptoms.

Staying active is also key to managing symptoms and staying healthy. Exercise can help improve energy levels, reduce pain, and boost your immune system. However, it's important to listen to your body and avoid overexertion. Gentle forms of exercise such as walking, yoga, and tai chi may be more appropriate for people with autoimmune diseases.

Finally, it's essential to work closely with your doctor and other healthcare professionals to manage symptoms and stay healthy. Regular check-ups and monitoring of symptoms can help catch potential issues early, and your doctor can make adjustments to your treatment plan as needed.

CONCLUSION

Taking control of your health is one of the most important steps you can take towards a fulfilling and healthy life. The impact of our health on our lives cannot be overstated – it affects our energy levels, our mood, our ability to do the things we love, and even our longevity. However, in today's fast-paced world, taking control of our health often takes a back seat to other priorities. With so many distractions, it can be difficult to focus on our health and wellness, but it is absolutely crucial that we do.

One of the main reasons why taking control of our health is so important is because it can help us to prevent serious health problems from developing in the first place. By living a healthy lifestyle and taking care of our bodies, we can reduce our risk of developing chronic diseases such as heart disease, diabetes, and cancer. By making healthy choices, such as eating a balanced diet, getting regular exercise, and avoiding harmful habits like smoking and excessive drinking, we can help our bodies to function at their best and protect ourselves from future health problems.

In addition to preventing serious health problems, taking control of our health can also help us to manage existing health conditions more effectively. For example, if you have been diagnosed with high blood pressure or high cholesterol, taking control of your health can help you to manage these conditions through lifestyle changes and medication, reducing your risk of serious complications such as heart attack or stroke.

One of the best ways to take control of your health is to work with a healthcare provider who can help you to create a customized plan for your specific health needs. Your healthcare provider can help you to identify any health risks that you may be facing, and can help you to create a plan to manage these risks effectively. They can also help you to understand how your lifestyle and habits may be affecting your health, and can give you advice on how to make positive changes that can help you to feel your best.

One of the most important steps you can take to take control of your health is to be proactive about your healthcare. This means making regular appointments with your healthcare provider, getting regular check-ups and screenings, and being proactive about monitoring your health. This may include monitoring your blood pressure, cholesterol levels, and blood sugar levels, as well as paying attention to any changes in your energy levels or mood. By being proactive about your healthcare, you can stay ahead of any health problems that may arise, and take steps to manage these problems effectively before they become more serious.

Another important aspect of taking control of your health is to make positive lifestyle changes that can have a major impact on your health and wellbeing. This may include making changes to your diet, such as reducing your intake of sugar, processed foods, and unhealthy fats, and increasing your intake of nutrient-rich fruits and vegetables. It may also include getting regular exercise, which can help you to maintain a healthy weight, reduce your risk of chronic diseases, and improve your mood and energy levels.